# Just Live It

*How to Optimize Your Health, Master Discipline, and Rise Above It All*

## BY

## George Farah, PHD

# JUST LIVE IT

Copyright © 2024 by George Farah.

All rights reserved. No part of this publication may be reproduced, distributed, or transmitted in any form or by any means, including photocopying, recording, or other electronic or mechanical methods, without the prior written permission of the author, except in the case of brief quotations embodied in critical reviews and certain other non-commercial uses permitted by copyright law.

Ordering Information: Special discounts are available on quantity purchases by corporations, associations, as well as U.S. trade bookstores and wholesalers.

www.DreamStartersPublishing.com

GEORGE FARAH, PHD

# Table of Contents

Introduction ..................................................................... 4
Discipline ........................................................................ 8
Mindset Mastery ........................................................... 15
Unearthing Your Purpose ............................................. 29
Embracing Consistency and the Value of Habits ......... 41
The Importance of Routine and Balance ..................... 54
Following The Natural Way ......................................... 66
Measurement, Management, and Enjoying the Journey ................. 81
Truth, Sacrifice, and the Lens of Clarity ...................... 88
Living Life with Purpose ............................................... 93
Be All In ....................................................................... 101
Money is Important, But It's Not Everything ............. 107
Prioritizing Health and Body Care .............................. 113
Guru ............................................................................ 120
Join Our Community .................................................. 124

JUST LIVE IT

# **Introduction**

---

In the hills of Lebanon, as the civil war raged and transformed the land I called home, I quickly learned that life was as unpredictable as it was precious. My childhood memories are painted with both vibrant tales of tradition and family, but not without the harsh realities of conflict and war time. But even in the face of such adversity, it was in those very hills that the roots of my unrelenting spirit were planted.

When I first came to this country thirty-five years ago, it was to chase the American dream. My aspirations were larger than my pockets, and I had to quickly tap into my survival mode mindset. With no other options available, I lived in my car and worked tireless hours scrubbing floors at a McDonald's. I believed with every fiber of my being that I would one day become one of the greatest bodybuilders in the world. I knew my life's story had to change, and it did.

On the rise to my bodybuilding stardom, when circumstances seemed like they were finally moving in a positive direction, I was shot. This wasn't just some flesh wound. I was shot three times by armed robbers. Before I knew it, burning hot sensations were coursing through my body. I thought I was done living in violent times when I made it to the States, and that I'd be safe to just stop at the store and grab a gallon of milk. But, as each bullet pierced into me, memories of friends and family whom I had lost started to come into focus, and I suddenly had a vivid experience of stepping into the light toward those loved ones.

It sounds like something you'd see in a movie—someone going toward the light—but that's what it was. Unexplainable things had happened to me, and although I'm still learning why, I realize that each experience has shaped me in ways I never could have imagined.

The lessons I learned from extraordinary experiences throughout my life have taught me things more valuable than any amount of money or championship titles ever could. Everything that's happened to me in my life has been a steppingstone, guiding me to the stage of the greatest bodybuilding competition in the world, Mr. Olympia in 2002, after which I would help coach over 130 different athletes to step on that very same stage.

With things looking up again, my journey still had more to teach me. In 2017, I faced an opponent fiercer than any bodybuilder (and my glory days of Ronnie Coleman and Jay Cutler). This opponent didn't play by the rules and had a plan more devious than anything imaginable—advanced, stage 3c colorectal cancer.

In spite of facing a quickly spreading cancer and succumbing to the odds, I turned to what I knew best: discipline, consistency, positivity, and unwavering commitment. Using my deep understanding of nutrition and holistic healing, I not only defeated my own cancer but went on to guide others on their paths to remission, as well.

The essence of my story is not one of pain or suffering but of transformation and rebirth. Each challenge I've faced has been an opportunity to grow stronger, to understand this beautiful life a little more, and to share my lessons and insights with the world. You don't have to be sick to read my book, you just have to be ready to grow.

I've learned that every negative can be flipped into a positive, every setback is a setup for a greater comeback, and the most potent fuel for anyone's journey is a strong, deeply rooted "why."

This book is a reflection of my life, but more importantly, it's an invitation for you to reexamine and be thankful for yours. It's an invitation to understand that the battles you face, the hardships you endure, and the number of times you get back up, are what define and strengthen you. It's a beacon for those in the throes of their darkest moments, offering hope and insight into how adversity, when approached with the right mindset, can be the catalyst for incredible change.

As you work your way through these pages, remember that life is not about avoiding the storms and the hard times. It's about having faith that you can weather them, and maybe even dance in the rain. Through my experiences, I hope to propel you to lead a healthier, more positive, and profoundly impactful life. Join me as we embark on this journey together. A journey of war, trials, and triumph.

# Chapter 1

# Discipline

**(The Foundation of Survival)**

---

*"In the realm of ideas, everything depends on enthusiasm; in the real world, all rests on perseverance."*

**Johann Wolfgang von Goethe, German poet and playwright**

I grew up amidst a civil war in my home country, where seeking shelter from bombs and gunfire, that not only caused deprivation of the land but to the very souls of the people, became the new normal. So was the feeling of fear.

Each day of survival from the mayhem and constant state of fear was considered a blessing, and we had to live them as if they were our last (because they might have been).

# GEORGE FARAH, PHD

Through every echoing gunshot, every hushed whisper of fear and danger, I didn't know then how positively this chaos would impact my life. It taught me how to survive, and thus, it taught me discipline.

Discipline isn't something you have or are born with. You have to harness the power of discipline, and for me, constantly being in a state of survival is what instilled that powerful trait within me. This wasn't the discipline to avoid your desserts now and then (although, that's not a bad idea either). This was the kind that kept my family and me alive.

There's something raw and real about discipline that evolves from a state of survival. When every decision is literally life or death, you quickly understand the value of focus, determination, and unwavering commitment. You appreciate all the small things and don't take them for granted. This lifestyle also teaches what you don't want out of this life and reinforces that you are meant for something greater.

I knew I was meant for something greater. While the surroundings of my youth were challenging, they laid the foundation for the discipline that I would harness in every venture of my life. This direction has saved my life more than once.

# JUST LIVE IT

## Juggling Dreams and Reality

Let's jump forward a few years to when I was on a relentless mission to become one of the greatest bodybuilders of all time. When I came to this land thirty-five years ago, I thought I was going to instantly start living the American dream. Boy, did I have some wakeup calls. At times, I would live out of my car, working two and sometimes three jobs just to make ends meet. And if that weren't enough, I would add night school on top of it. If you've never lived out of your car, let me tell you, it is a rough and dangerous way to live. However, I was determined to fulfill my potential for greatness. I was surer than anything that my efforts would be rewarded. With my tired eyes, aching muscles, and the ever-present lure of a comfortable bed after a grueling shift, I persisted. That same discipline that had seen me through the perils of war now fueled my hunger and ambition.

I remember those nights, and I'm grateful for them. Wanting to do nothing but sleep, I'd push through another lecture, finish that last homework assignment, then show up for work. Whether I realized it or not, I was instilling some of the strictest rules and guidelines for myself. I didn't know this was the real life of an entrepreneur; I just knew what I had to do to continue on for one more day.

Every single one of these choices—the choice to sacrifice what I wanted now for what I wanted to achieve later—was driven by my overarching "why." My "why" was my compass. It was my North Star that never led me astray, no matter how rough things got. I wasn't just chasing a degree, paycheck, or a bed (although, a soft mattress would've been nice a little sooner). I was chasing a dream, a better future, and every small step was a part of that larger journey.

## Discipline in Adversity

Throughout this book, we will dive deeper into certain parts of my life. But I will tell you a bit about maintaining structure when life throws you the nastiest of curveballs. In 2017, I was diagnosed with stage 3c colorectal cancer. Stage 3c is right before stage 4, which is when the cancer spread all over the body. At this point, my mindset was ironclad, my clarity on my life's purpose was crystal clear, and I believed that everything was positive. Stage 3c? Fine, but I knew my story wasn't ending there.

My first surgery to remove the tumor attached to my intestines and bladder lasted twelve hours. This was followed by a few other surgeries for numerous complications. I will tell you now that I think that removing my gallbladder was one of the biggest mistakes of my life.

Before going in for the surgeries, the doctors told me it was necessary because the cancer had spread locally. With my knowledge and background in nutrition, I decided to try things my way rather than big pharma's way. Not that I didn't think the doctors meant well, but when it came to nutrition, I trusted myself with that more than them.

I'm not here to try to provide medical advice or say this is how you should eat if you have cancer, but this is what worked for *me*. I went on a mostly vegan diet with no animal proteins and stuck to whole foods. I avoided anything that was processed, full of sugar, or just unnatural. And in a room full of chemo patients, who bore the ravages of treatments, I was the only one who didn't lose his hair. Not only that, but I was also putting weight on when most struggle to do that. I was working out regularly, eating clean, and felt great for a guy being on chemotherapy.

Meanwhile, the clinic was giving other people bologna sandwiches, pizza, candy, and pretty much anything to try to get them to gain weight. Little did they know that these foods were only going to make those people sicker, if not lead them to their death beds.

In cancer patients, doctors and nurses will monitor what's known as your CA-125 levels. Normal ranges for people fall between 0-35 U/ml (units per milliliter). Before any surgeries, I got mine down to zero within five months of my diagnosis. Five months, some chemo and radiation, and a healthy diet and lifestyle. Not just within normal ranges, but at 0. As you can probably guess, the doctors were asking me what I did. Then, before long, the food they were giving their patients during treatments had changed to beans and other whole foods that were well-sourced and going to actually make a difference.

Food is the best medicine in the world. You just need to listen to your body when it starts to tell you something is going wrong, or when it's going right.

## The Choices We Make

As we progress through my journey and this book, you will find that my discipline was not just about doing what was needed, it was about recognizing when to pivot and when to stay the course. Just because things got tough didn't mean I was going down the wrong path for me. People quit when things get tough, and that's why most never accomplish what they'd hoped or set out to do. Every phase, every challenge, taught me something invaluable. If I could see the regimen in a bodybuilder, I knew they had the mettle for challenges beyond the gym. That's the kind of order I respect, and those are the people I'd always want by my side.

# Takeaways

1. **Identify your "why."** Spend some time introspecting and understanding your purpose. What drives you? What's the bigger picture you're working toward?

## JUST LIVE IT

Having clarity on this will make your path of discipline more navigable. Your why and purpose are your guiding light. With whatever you do in life, you need to have a sense of direction and purpose. Otherwise, we just drift along and, before we know it, we're on a death bed, wondering what we actually did with our lives.

2. **Find a way to keep yourself disciplined.** Whether it's a physical journal or an app, track your daily disciplines. It could be as simple as drinking enough water, avoiding certain foods, or dedicating time to a hobby. Monitoring these will reinforce your commitment and show you tangible progress.
3. **Have daily affirmations.** Start or end your day with affirmations. As it would align with this chapter, Jocko Willink has coined the mantra that, "Discipline equals freedom." Let it be a daily reminder that each act of discipline is a step closer to the life you aspire to lead. Discipline will get you farther than motivation ever will. Discipline is about doing what needs to be done when you don't want to do it.

# Chapter 2

# Mindset Mastery

## (The Drive to Lead)

---

*"Your beliefs become your thoughts, your thoughts become your words, your words become your actions, your actions become your habits, your habits become your values, your values become your destiny."*

**Mahatma Gandhi, Indian lawyer and ethicist**

In the heat of Lebanon, particularly during war times, every dawn was like a fresh slate. A new day, a new chance, a new beginning. The day was mine to own or be owned by it.

Watching my father work as hard as he did, I learned from an early age that if I wanted something in this life, I was going to have to earn it. No one was going to give it to me.

Who was I? The world is so large, with so many people of a similar mindset. I knew I had my work cut out for me, but hard work was nothing that I was going to shy away from. I saw my father work hard my entire life. He was an entrepreneur who sold stockings. Man, he was a salesman. He could sell candy to a bodybuilder in prep. Unfortunately, it was during the war that everything was burned, leaving him with nothing. But I saw a man who never gave up and fought for it all. So, that's how I knew how to operate, and that was a good start.

## Seeking Opportunities Over Handouts

Before landing in America, I always envisioned how great it would be as soon as I got here. I'd constantly think, "Wow, look at them." What couldn't you do in America? But coming to America was hard for me. I had to learn English pretty fast, because all I knew was Arabic and French at the time. It's good to be able to speak multiple languages, but English was a tough one to pick up! I knew it was part of what it would take and muscled through it, anyway.

Fortunately, my brother and his wife already lived here, in Tucson, Arizona. They agreed to take me in for a while until I found my footing a bit.

My first job was selling furniture. Turns out I had picked a few things up from my old man, watching him sell stockings.

# GEORGE FARAH, PHD

I wasn't too bad, either! Over the course of three half days of work, my first check came in the amount of $60. That might not sound like much, but for my first job in America, it was a big deal.

I had borrowed my brother's car that day to get to work, and I got pulled over for speeding on the way home. That had never happened to me before. So, needless to say, I was a bit nervous. The officer was really nice to me, but not nice enough to not write me a ticket. When I saw the amount that I had to pay, a wave of defeat came over me. $60 speeding ticket. The exact amount of what I had just earned working at the furniture store.

Welp, back to square one.

Now, a speeding ticket isn't that big of a deal, but I didn't want to give my brother and his wife any unwanted or unnecessary trouble. So, I decided that Arizona wasn't for me. Of course, they were very adamant that I could stay as long as I needed in order for me to get my feet back under me, but I wanted to make my own way. I decided to try my luck in Chicago. I had a friend who had been living there, and he offered to let me crash with him for a while until I was able to start making some money and find my own place. At the time, I started working at McDonald's as a cook. I would work, go home to get whatever type of workout I could come up with,

## JUST LIVE IT

eat, sleep, and do it all over again the next day. I luckily found work, a place to live, and a routine. It was only a matter of time before everything else started to fall into place. Or so I thought …

Now, obviously money was tight, but I would buy whatever healthy foods I could at the store, and when possible, just strictly eat some protein at work, which was usually okay. I mean, we did get a discount; might as well use it, right?

I've found that, oftentimes, we need to watch what else is being added to our proteins. Are all meats bad? Maybe, maybe not. But when you read about how bad some foods are, it's important to look at what is being paired with it. Are you eating a steak lathered in butter? Is your chicken breast covered in alfredo sauce on top of a bunch of pasta? French fries or fake cheese slices on top of your hamburger? We kind of all know, more or less, what's healthier and what's not. Some need more guidance than others but think about getting as close to the natural form of the food as possible. But we'll get way deeper into the nutrition weeds later in the book, because I have some crazy stories on healing sick people just by fixing their food …

At this point, I was getting in better and better shape, to the point that I started to turn some heads. I was getting deeper knowledge in nutrition and training research, with the goal to make some waves in the fitness industry.

While at my McDonald's job, the manager was one of these turned heads. She started to take a liking to me, so much so that I had to deny the pass she made toward me. At work, in the middle of the shift, I'm trying to toss some fries while she's trying to do a lot more than take people's food orders. Unfortunately, she took this pretty personally because, the next day, I was the new janitor. Brother can't even work without getting in trouble.

Not only did my boss give me the boot, but our landlord found out about two of us living in a studio apartment, and he didn't like that. So, instead of trying to find a new place in Chicago, I decided to move to Rochester, New York. Another friend was kind enough to take me in while I found my footing, but that didn't last long once I found out he was selling drugs. So far, the "American dream" was more elusive to me than I was to my McDonald's manager.

## Developing a Bulletproof Mindset

No way was I going to risk the troubles that came with living under the same roof as a drug dealer. I just got to America and didn't want to get caught up in all that. Hell, I didn't want any more speeding tickets, let alone being an accessory to dealing drugs.

That was when I lived out of my car for a while. I see people almost treat that act as some sort of entrepreneurial martyrdom. It's not. It's a dangerous lifestyle that should be a last resort. However, it teaches you a lot. It teaches you the place that you never want to be again and will ignite a spark in you that very few others in the world can relate to. My mindset and mentality aren't the stereotypical "get shit done" that you see all over the internet.

Mine comes from survival.

Trust me; I didn't want to live in my car and bounce around, but I knew the environment and things that would be most conducive for me, and I was searching for a solid foothold to grow my life in America. I went through these hardships over and over because I needed to. I had to survive, and I wasn't about to try to take a shortcut. Although, I do understand how people can turn to selling drugs or trying to make some fast money. It's attractive when you think you have no other option. When you don't see a way out and all roads point to easy money. I'll tell you right now, there's no such thing as fast, easy money that's legal. Unless you win the lottery, that cash is dangerous. It can either cause you to get arrested or get scammed and lose everything. Plus, I think struggle is good and more people need to experience some harsher parts of it.

Think about my perspective. To me, living in my car in America is still better than worrying about where missiles, mortars, and gunfire were going to strike on any given day. I grew up in war. I can make it living out of my car for a while.

Survival.

By this point, I was about twenty-two, maybe twenty-three years old. I had finally gotten a job as a security guard at a hair extension and accessory parlor. The owners were Jewish, knew my story, and were so kind to take me in and allow me to work for them. Although they couldn't pay me a whole lot, they paid what they could but taught me even more.

You know, it's interesting. We read and watch the news about all the wars and unfortunate happenings around the world right now. People at odds due to land and religion, and those who say certain cultures can or can't co-exist. The Jewish owners of the shop and I built a relationship on *who* the other person was, not *what.* We all worked hard, all good people, all trying to make it, and each of us wanting to help the other advance in this crazy life. That was it. No ulterior motive or sinister feeling toward the other. That was the first time I really felt the power of "the land of opportunity."

Along with working as a security guard at the parlor, I was a bouncer at a nightclub. From all my time already spent in the gym, I was enough of a presence to get those jobs relatively easier than anything else.

Between both jobs, I was finally able to afford my own place to live, and even started going to a New York community college. And it wouldn't be topped off without confirming I got myself a gym membership. My heart and vision never lost sight of the long-term goal of making my mark on the fitness industry. I was merely going through all the steppingstones necessary to get there.

Throughout all the speed bumps, I always took the negative and turned it into a positive. If you focus on nothing but bad things, that is what will come. When you constantly focus on the good things, then that is what you will be blessed with. I'm not saying you won't have to go through the hard things for a while, but stay focused on the good, your overall goal, and I promise that you will come out the other end victorious.

## Embracing Continued Learning Through Challenges

It's clear that I got my entrepreneurial spirit from my father. He was the epitome of what a father and role model should be. You hear all the time that kids watch way more than they listen. That's exactly what I did. I saw my dad work hard for his family day in and day out. I saw him struggle when his entire inventory of stockings was burned and gone forever. And throughout it all, he showed the way to turn a negative into a positive and to keep pushing forward. Inventory burned. Okay, now what is he going to do about it?

Over time, the owners of the parlor and I became quite close. Sure, I worked for them, but we were friends. We were all immigrants who came to America in search of a better life, so we looked out for each other.

One day, they came in and told me that their daughter had been in a car accident. She was okay, but the car was going to be totaled. Thinking about more ways to make money, I asked how much they wanted for it. They sold it to me, and every few days, I would work on the car in an attempt to fix it up. At first, it was just about needing my own car. But after working on that car and becoming pretty good at it, I realized this could be a whole business with pretty good returns.

The next day, I bought practically every newspaper I could find because people would post cars for sale in the ads section. Before I knew it, I had a really good side gig going on. After acquiring a few cars, I found a body shop that I could pay the owner a few bucks to fix and clean them up. That became my main spot for fixing all the cars and was turning a tidy profit on each vehicle, so much so that I was able to quit my nightclub job and focus a bit more on school.

It's funny how everything ends up being connected. Each little steppingstone led to something bigger and better, even if I didn't see it or think it at the time. If it weren't for the parlor owners allowing me to be their security guard (and me willing to work for cheap), then I wouldn't have bought the damaged car and realized I was pretty good at fixing and flipping them. This would eventually lead to me opening my own car lot around the age of twenty-two or twenty-three. I was hooked on entrepreneurship. I knew that I could never sit behind a desk all day for work. I liked being out and doing things, creating something, and watching the fruits of my labor grow.

At that time, I was making a lot of money with my car lot. After a while, a friend of mine was selling cell phones (this was when they were barely becoming a hot commodity). He would sell entire plans and make an absolute killing on them. I figured, why not build an empire and get in on the action?

The nightclub I used to bounce at was my first stop since I still had good relations with them. When you're a regular nightclub goer and see someone else have the first cell phone, it creates a frenzy. I was selling plans for $350 and throwing in the actual phone for free.

Someone else caught onto this business model, and his competition just about drove me bankrupt. Remember, I was in Rochester, New York. At a certain point, there's only so much space! Fortunately, I was able to sell the remainder of my inventory to a guy in Mexico and got out fairly unscathed.

My next venture was quite a scandal. Literally. After being successful at buying and flipping cars, I started doing the same with houses. I linked up with a crew who seemed pretty legit doing some major deals and projects. What happened, though, was that I would front the money for the houses, sign off on all the paperwork, and technically be liable for the physical structures. The rest of the crew would do their jobs, the house would sell, but I wouldn't see any of the profits. So, I was left with all the houses and no money.

I wasn't their first victim in this scam. As a matter of fact, they were doing this on such a large scale that the FBI had to get involved. Their whole operation scammed people out of a total of $60 million! Of course, I didn't see any of my money again. The head of the scam ended up dying in prison, and I went bankrupt.

Within a couple years of being in America, I had lived in three cities, gotten a speeding ticket, kicked out of one place, lived with a drug dealer in another, lived out of my car, started night school, opened multiple successful businesses, and gone bankrupt. Welcome to the "American dream."

# Creating Leaders Through Shared Experiences

To say life is a journey would be quite an understatement. But that's exactly what it is. Each one of us has our own unique path to follow, and each path has its own detours and ups and downs. But by sharing my stories, the wins and losses, I hope to illuminate a path for those looking to blaze their own trail. Hopefully, you can step on a few less landmines than I did, or at least not the same ones. If I can relate to and help even a single person navigate their journey and have a better life, then my hardships and lessons learned will be more than worth it. It's through the sharing of experiences that we not only find common ground but can inspire leadership in one another, as well.

From the chaotic streets of Lebanon to the restless Windy City, and finally landing in the cold nights of Rochester, my journey had been nothing short of a roller coaster. And we're just getting warmed up! Each city, job, and challenge left a permanent impression on me and taught me lessons that would eventually mold me into the man I am today. And while I faced some different struggles, these experiences weren't just about me. They became tales to tell of resilience and determination, in hopes of inspiring another generation of entrepreneurs and go-getters.

This book is more than just a recounting of my life. It's to inspire others in a similar position to do something similar: share your story. Doing so is a different way to extend a helping hand, a mentorship from afar, with the ability to help people with indirect contact. Every leader, entrepreneur, bodybuilder, or writer can connect, inspire, and foster more leaders in this world.

So, I implore others to learn from my stories, let them guide you, and then share your own with someone else. Together, we can create a world of inspired leaders and workers, ready to make a difference.

## Takeaways

1. **Take risks.** Moving to a different state or city, let alone another country, is tough. It's scary. But it allows you to have a fresh start and also prove things to yourself. Even if I weren't in a war-torn country, I'd want to visit different places and cultures and simply learn new things. There's the saying that "fortune favors the bold." In the simplest terms, think about admirable entrepreneurs, athletes, you name it; one of the things they all have in common is that they all took risks. You don't become the best by staying comfortable. If you want to be the best, you have to compete against and beat the best. That's quite a risk, but it's always going to be worth the attempt.
2. **Learn through your challenges.** We're all going to face hard times and challenges, whether you take infinitely more risks than someone else or not. It's just a part of life. What you do with it, now that's a different

story. I encourage you to soak in your next big hurdle or loss and try to find the value in it. It might not make itself present at first but open your mind to the fact that there could be some blessing in disguise in why that particular thing happened. As I mentioned before, I always turn a negative into a positive. Many times, that's easier said than done. But when you start to get in the habit of it, your entire outlook and response to tough situations becomes so much better.

3. **Share your experiences.** It's important to help your fellow men/women. Sharing your stories sounds like a simple act (because it is), but it can have profound effects on helping guide others through their own journey. You never know which random story or lesson learned might resonate with someone else in a similar position. From something you said to an actionable response to a problem, the more you share, the better.

# Chapter 3

# Unearthing Your Purpose

*"Don't ask what the world needs. Ask what makes you come alive, and go do it. Because what the world needs is people who have come alive."*

**Howard Thurman, American writer and philosopher**

In this crazy game of life, people often get confused that our accomplishments are what define us. But it's more than that. It's about our reasons for pursuing such grandiose agendas. Our motivations, our inner compass, that's what fuels the fire for our life journey. And it's these pursuits that can resonate with others and inspire future generations.

# JUST LIVE IT

When we speak of ambition, passion, and drive, it all circles back to our deeply rooted "why." Our "why" is about discovering purpose and using it to change the contours of an entire industry. So many people are lost in this world, and it typically stems from a lack of purpose, fulfillment, and direction. If we all had a clear mission, and even a rough plan of that mission, then I think we would see a lot of people and society in a very different place.

## The Power of a Transformative "Why"

In 1997, my life took a drastic turn. While stopping at the store with my friends to get some milk, I was shot three times with .45 hollow-point bullets. An armed robbery gone awry. Those hollow points changed the direction of my life, when they were meant to end it. I was pronounced dead. And for a minute, I thought I was. There was the light that you'll hear those reference to when people have had a near death experience. Or what will be described in just about any movie with a similar scenario. I was headed toward this bright, white light, and soon, it surrounded me.

Slowly, people from my past started to appear. Family and friends, most of whom had died as a result of the war in Lebanon. Then everyone started to guide me in another direction. Soon, I was able to make out what it was they were all walking me toward: a coffin. Before I knew it, the lid of the coffin was closing and everyone in my vision seemed to give me a look of peace and comfort.

Already being claustrophobic, I wasn't having some lid closed on me. I pushed my hands up against the top of the coffin and woke up at the very same moment the doctors were shocking me back to life. God wasn't done with me yet. If He was, that would have been the time for me to go home to Him. There was a lot more to my "why" that had to be fulfilled.

Once I recovered from the shooting, it was game on. My fitness and nutrition were on point in no time. I would spend the next couple years dialing in every facet of my training and nutrition, and I eventually signed up for a show. After winning the first, I started to gain even more traction for my training business and had a lot of people coming in the doors of Samson Powerhouse Gym. After a while, I figured it was time to try to obtain my pro card.

For those who don't know, obtaining an IFBB (International Federation of Bodybuilding) Pro card is one of the highest accolades in the world of bodybuilding. Outside of winning on some of the world's biggest stages, becoming a pro is definitely something to write home about. Even if you don't make it much farther past that, getting to that point emphasizes the level of discipline, dedication, hard work, and sacrifice that very few would ever understand.

To give you a reference, only about five to six people each year become bodybuilding professionals. You become

## JUST LIVE IT

licensed at an elite level where you are able to compete against the best of the best. Turning pro says you're about that life, and you're here to make a mark. So, in 2001, when the time came for me to register for a show where I could qualify to become pro, I was pretty confident going in. Not cocky, but highly confident in my hard work, knowledge, and ability to look the absolute best on stage.

A few weeks before the show, I made a business card that read:

*IFBB Pro: George Farah*

That's it. Nothing more. When I arrived at the facility, I found the judges and gave each of them a business card. They, knowing I was there to try to get my card but not yet a pro, had a good laugh. Of course, they thought, "Who does this guy think he is?" But I knew how I looked, how conditioned I was, and I felt great in every facet of the word. Mentally, physically, and spiritually, I was ready.

If something in your life is off or going wrong, it's going to show on stage. There's no two ways around it. If you're really stressed, it'll show. If you're not right with people or things in your life, it's all going to come out. Stepping on that stage and posing in a little bathing suit for complete strangers is one of the most vulnerable situations you can put yourself in. If you're not right, everyone will know. But that wasn't me. Stare at me in my swimsuit. I'm here to win the damn thing.

At these types of bodybuilding shows, there are "callouts." That's where judges call out a certain number of athletes to determine the rank of each, particularly when some athletes are very close in the points.

When it was time for callouts, I didn't hear my name. It took a quick second, but I realized that they didn't call my name because they needed to see who would fight for second and third place. I had blown away everyone to the point that they didn't need to see me pose anymore. I won and earned the title of IFBB Pro.

Once I got back to the gym, the owner, James Raquel, gave me a free membership. I told him that wasn't necessary, but he insisted. The amount of people I already brought into the gym before the show was significant, but that number grew immensely after I became a pro, and I could barely keep up. He saw the value of how much exposure his gym was getting and figured a free gym membership for me was the least he could do. At this point, money wasn't an issue, but lowering any cost is always nice!

From then on, I had phone calls, emails, and walk-ins coming to me twenty-four seven to try to train with me. I was finally fulfilling the "why" that I had set out for myself.

# JUST LIVE IT

## Insights from an Expert

Simon Sinek is an author and motivational speaker in the area of business leadership. He's observed everyone from Navy SEALs to the highest performing CEOs in an effort to figure out some of the biggest key components that drive an individual through his or her life, as well as the decisions they make.

According to Sinek, the "why" behind any business or business model is not solely making money. Although that is a very important piece to any and every business, that usually is not the strongest "why" that one can have. Rather, he points to a cause, vision, or purpose. Something that is deeply rooted in the very fabric of a person's being.

An organization or individual's "why" is what inspires action. It's what gets people bought into the mission, or not. But when someone else shares that vision, they feel compelled to act because it is now a part of their purpose, as well. When an emotional connection is created between the worker and the business's work being done, you're bound to have a great employee and work culture.

It's not about what you do but why you do it, and mine was fairly simple. I wanted to help others to the best of my abilities, and I found myself being really good at anything related to fitness. I had a knack for it, and then that turned into tangible results. Eventually, it became the only thing I wanted to do.

I sank all of myself into this mission, and here I am. It was about helping people as much as I can, the best way I know how, and then sharing those experiences and insights with the rest of the world.

The graph below is a simple illustration of Simon Sinek's that encapsulates this whole notion. He talks about acting, thinking, and communicating in the most effective way possible: from the inside out.

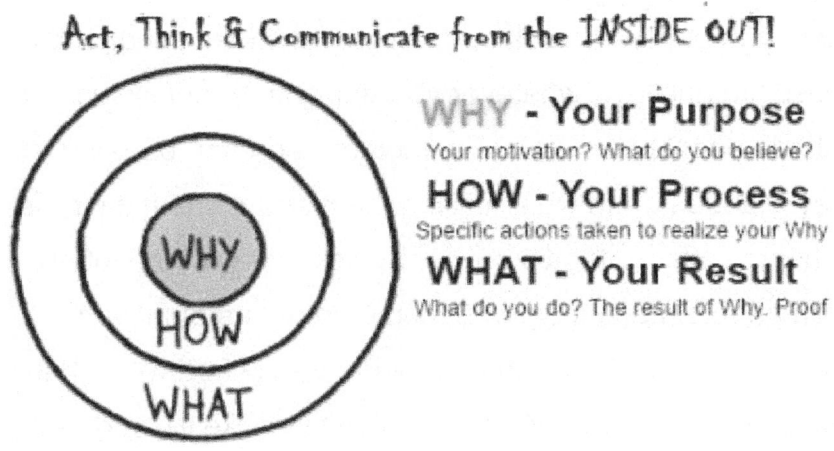

Photo: Simon Sinek, Start With Why.

As you can see, your "what" is the result. What do you do? What is the final outcome of the decision? Then you have the "how." That's the process of the thing you are trying to accomplish. These are your specific actions that it will take to realize the actualize "why." And at the center of it all, the true driving force behind what and how you are doing the thing, is your "why," your purpose and motivation. What do you believe? What is your reasoning for doing the thing you're doing? Having a clear drive of purpose and fulfillment and following what you believe you're called to do on this earth, it can be the strongest guide for your life. Many people are lost in this world, but digging deep to understand your why and purpose can change your entire outlook and approach to your life.

Do you want to know the power of having a strong, deeply rooted "why?" Look at any person of great success whom you admire or look up to. It can be in anything: acting, fitness, technology, whatever your thing is. Every single one of those people was driven by their mission and purpose. They grabbed on to what fulfilled them and made it their fuel for how to attack life. It's not some lucky draw of the lottery when people make it big or become someone of influence. They were consistent with their work, disciplined with what had to be done (even when they didn't feel like it), and had an absolute desire for that thing they chased.

## Writing to Inspire, Not Just to Inform

This is a lot more than slapping some ink on a page. It's my heart, soul, blood, and tears from my life experiences. I didn't pick up the pen (or open the laptop) to become a bestselling author. I wrote to inspire change and share some of the most impactful life lessons I've learned over the years. This book is my legacy and a way of reaching out to anyone who might be on the brink of giving up or feeling lost on their journey.

For me, every person I trained, from the great Dwayne "The Rock" Johnson to the hundred plus athletes who graced the Olympia stage, was a testament of purpose. It always thrilled me to see those people grow, both in their physical and personal journeys. But more than that, it was about creating a bond and camaraderie that went beyond the confines of the gym.

In my years as a trainer, I've been more blessed with the people who came to work with me. It's so humbling to be the man behind the curtain, helping them prepare for some of the biggest events of their lives. But with every single individual, they all knew their "why." They felt called to something bigger than themselves and had a sense of purpose. That inner compass for them was guiding them in a single direction and they were laser focused on getting to their destination.

When you have people who set a goal, it makes my job a whole lot easier. I can't figure out their reasoning for them; that's their job. And whether most of them knew this or not, it

# JUST LIVE IT

wasn't just about the trophies, the bragging rights, or the clout. It was about the transformation.

When you're that driven and motivated to accomplish a task, it is so much easier to stick to a plan. So many times, I see people who wander through the gym, curious what exercise they should do next, without a clear goal in mind just for that day, let alone the next sixteen to twenty weeks.

If there's one thing I hope you take away from this book, it's the understanding that your purpose is the most powerful tool you possess. It's the flame that will light your way through the darkest of times, the compass that will guide you when you're lost and unsure of where to go or what to do next. Embrace it, nurture it, and let it drive you toward your dreams. Even if it takes you in directions you never thought were going to be a part of your journey, sometimes those detours help you get closer to your goals than you think. Who knows, they might even show something different that you want to pursue and never thought possible.

When I think back to those early days in America, moving from city to city, job to job, I recognize that every challenge, every adversity, was a blessing in disguise. And often times, our hardships have blessings hidden within them. We just have to be open-minded enough to accept and look for them.

These lessons were not just for me, but they became stories that I could share with the rest of the world, in hopes that someone somewhere could benefit from them. Whether it was the pride of earning my first paycheck at the furniture store or the resilience I discovered in myself after being shot or diagnosed with cancer, each story carries its own seed of wisdom.

Together, we can discover the power of purpose, the strength that comes from understanding one's true calling, and the spirit of the human heart. With every story, every lesson, I hope to empower you to chase your dreams with the same passion and determination that fueled my journey. This book isn't a simple recounting of events, but an invitation, a call to look within and discover your "why," and embark on a journey filled with passion, purpose, and promise. Remember, every challenge is an opportunity, every setback a lesson. Embrace each and every one of them, learn from them, and let them propel you toward your destiny. The world awaits your unique story; all you have to do is have the courage to write it.

## **<u>Takeaways</u>**

1. **Discover your why.** Every endeavor, dream, and challenge becomes surmountable when powered by a strong "why." It's not enough to merely know what you're doing or how you're doing it. Dive deep into your soul and discover the reason you wake up each

morning. Is it for your family? A dream? A legacy? Knowing your "why" will act as an anchor, giving you direction during turbulent times and a reason to push forward when challenges arise.

2. **The transformative power of resilience.** Life will undoubtedly throw you curveballs, sometimes powerful enough to knock us off our feet. Yet, it's our ability to stand back up, just like I did after being shot and pronounced dead, which defines our character. Resilience isn't just about survival; it's about thriving and using adversities as steppingstones toward greatness.

3. **Inspire through actions, not just words.** It's easy to speak about change, passion, and goals. But true inspiration is birthed from actions. Whether it's writing a book, becoming a renowned bodybuilder, or being a beacon of hope for someone, let your deeds speak volumes. Remember, by living your truth and walking your path with integrity, you unconsciously permit others to do the same.

# Chapter 4

# Embracing Consistency and the Value of Habits

*"Success is neither magical nor mysterious. Success is the natural consequence of consistently applying basic fundamentals."*

**Jim Rohn, American entrepreneur, and writer**

In every task or venture that I've undertaken, whether it was building my physique, coaching others to reach their full potential, or building my business, there has always been one common thread woven throughout: consistency. It's what separates the ones who "make it" versus the ones who don't. There's a group that quits and a group that does what has to be done, even when they don't feel like it, and they keep pushing until the job is finished. Typically, however, those creator types never stop. They get a taste of what that consistency did for them, and building things becomes the new addiction. They have seen that the thing *can* work out, so they keep making new and better things happen. But above all else, they stay consistent.

## The Power of Consistency

Consistency is like the slow, steady heartbeat that keeps your dreams alive. It's a reaffirmation of commitment, an act of faith in the face of doubt, or lack of desire or want to accomplish the task at hand. In the world of entrepreneurship, this unwavering discipline and dedication is what separates those who make it and those who don't. It's the difference between, "Must be nice" and, "I built this." Everyone and their mother has an idea, a passion, some venture that is the next best thing. But very few actually stay the course, and it's those few who get to leave their mark on the world and live a life others will only dream of and look at from afar.

At the very start of something new, you have that initial spark of excitement that might keep you going a few weeks, maybe even a few months. But as things slowly unfold, that spark starts to fade. That's when the rest has to kick in. It's like the honeymoon stage in a new intimate relationship. Eventually, you choose to love that person, or you don't.

Entrepreneurship is similar. You choose to keep moving forward with what you started, or you quit.

In either scenario, it's not always fun and full of sunshine and rainbows. It is inevitable that you will fight with your significant other, and there will be times when you want to throw your computer against the wall and go back to a job where you can clock in, clock out, collect a consistent check and benefits, and call it a day.

Consistency isn't glamorous; it's a grind. But if you really want to achieve your dreams, you have to be obsessed with the beautiful grind.

There's a guy I know in sales and that was his favorite thing to tell his team. They specialize in window replacement, and the junior partners would canvas homes, looking at locations, how the house is kept and maintained, how visible it is from the street, how many windows you can see from the street, everything that might go into being the prime house for their windows.

The junior partners would drive around to prime areas, and when they found a good-looking house, they would knock on the door and try to set up an appointment with the homeowner(s) and the senior partner, who would do the actual selling of the windows. The better set up by the junior

# JUST LIVE IT

partner, the easier it becomes for the senior partner, and the more likely the job is to sell.

That work is an absolute grind, but it can also be highly rewarding and extremely lucrative. The guys who were consistently knocking on at least ten houses a day, improving their pitch and skills, and learning everything they could to become better, were the ones who performed the best in the office. That job is a grind. They're entrepreneurs.

There's a phrase that's fitting for entrepreneurship: "Gritty, not pretty." Because, a lot of times, it's not about who has the fanciest things or does things the prettiest way, but who has the most grit and is the most consistent.

Instagram shows that once you decide to be an entrepreneur, it's all private jets and Lamborghinis. Nuh-uh. Those things are possible, sure. But there is a workload, slew of sleepless nights, abundance of stress, blood, sweat, and tears that rarely gets shown. Anything is possible, but you had better bring your lunch, because you're going to have to earn every single thing you want in this game. You will be rewarded in many more ways than material things, but you have to be willing to go through the fire to get there.

Throughout my years in America, from the early days in Arizona to the bustling life in Chicago and then to Rochester, there were countless times when things got tough. I remember days when I barely made ends meet. Working at McDonald's, cleaning floors, living out of my car—I've been at

## GEORGE FARAH, PHD

the bottom. I know what it's like. Any of the roadblocks and adversities I faced could have easily discouraged any young immigrant trying to make it in a new country. But I never let go, never lost hope, and never lost faith in myself and my abilities. Every day, I reminded myself of why I had started and where I wanted to be. It wasn't just about making it through the day, but about building a life worth living.

Entrepreneurship is a marathon, not a sprint. Many businesses start with great promise, but quickly fade away. 90% of all startups fail. If you look at ten new businesses, one of them will succeed. Now, most of those 90% will likely survive the first year, but 70% of them will fail within the next five years. So, if you can make it to five years, then you're doing something right and might even have a chance at really making it.

One of the leading causes of these failures is a misinterpretation of the market demand. Just because you create it, doesn't mean people want it and will buy it. You need to do research and understand if what you want to sell is wanting to be bought. But if you start getting momentum, then you have to deliver results. Your earliest customers are your most important because they will either sing your praises or you'll just be another "nice guy who means well." You need to execute.

Early on in my training career, I was a walking billboard for my business. I walked the walk and practiced what I preached. But I also produced results for my clients, from me turning pro, to then helping others turn pro, and eventually coaching people to the Olympia stage. When I showed that I could get people to the biggest bodybuilding stage in the world, then there was no question about my abilities. So much so that I got the attention of Dwayne "The Rock" Johnson.

"The Rock" wanted *me* to train *him*. Produce consistent results, and there's no telling where it can lead.

But I will tell you one thing, those who win and create winners get recognized by others of the same caliber. Dwayne wasn't my first client. He came after hundreds of clients with consistent results. I didn't set out hoping to train celebrities. I set out with the goal of helping people, and I was in it for the long haul. I was prepared for the marathon I was about to take on. It's that kind of mindset that will take you farther than you ever thought possible.

## Shiny Object Syndrome

Too many times, people get caught up in the shiny object syndrome. Everyone wants everything *right now*. They want to be in shape after one week of working out and eating right. They want to be millionaires after one year. It doesn't work that way. There are extreme cases in business where something takes off, but that's just not how it works for most people. You have to commit and be ready to be in it for a long time, and you need to truly love and obsess over what you're going after. If not, you'll never make it.

This shiny object syndrome might sound familiar after I describe it in some more detail. This is a trait I've mostly seen in those trying to be successful in entrepreneurship, so we'll use some common ventures for examples. It only makes sense to start with personal training. Someone tries to become a full-time personal trainer on their own and build their own training business. Love it.

When they first start, they enter the stage of "Uninformed Optimism." This is where you're excited about the new venture, you're into the subject matter, super motivated, and you believe in yourself. There are tons of people doing this successfully, so surely you can, too.

The next stage is "Informed Pessimism." Here, you start learning the ins and outs of the business and realize there's a whole lot more than just telling people you're a trainer and training a few clients. This actually might be a little tougher than you thought, and now you're not sure if it will work out or if you can even get as far as finding out. A little doubt suddenly starts to creep in.

Then you hit what is famously known as the "Valley of Despair." It finally becomes apparent how much work this is actually going to take. Late nights, early mornings, lots of exhausting days, plenty of frustrations, lost time and money. You start to get blinded by everything that's going wrong and

## JUST LIVE IT

how hard it's going to be. You decide it's too much work and you're just going to keep your eye out for the next hot thing. You missed the ticket on this one, but you won't miss the prime time to get in at the next opportunity.

Let's break here for a second. This is the point that people give up. You get into the weeds of it all, and the tiniest things go wrong, and it scares you away from what you just said was your dream job. A little hardship, and you let your dream go just like that? Come on. If you can be run off that easily, it wasn't your thing to begin with. Any of you reading this are tougher than that. I might not know you personally, but I do know that. You're here because you're ready for change, and you're hungry for it. But if you can push through this valley of despair, where it seems like the odds are stacked against you, you will find yourself in a life-changing position. If you push through and tackle one thing at a time, one day at a time, you will start to see the tides change and the momentum start to pick up.

If you push through, you reach "Informed Optimism." You made it through the valley of despair. It's clear this is going to be harder than you thought at times, but it is possible and you are getting the hang of it. You're actually starting to take action and create a semi-functioning business. You start to get your confidence back, and you're excited again. You decide you're in it for the long haul.

# GEORGE FARAH, PHD

The last stage, the one that will set you up for life, is "Success and Fulfillment." It's working. You have a full-time training business. Maybe you have an employee or two, or maybe you have a consistently full schedule of clients. Either way, you've hit some major milestones. Take a minute to enjoy this moment. As an entrepreneur, there will always be another venture, another thing that looks like easy, fast money. There will always be shiny objects that will try to take you off your main course. Don't let it.

So many people try to do every single thing when, in reality, it's best if you stay focused on your one main thing. Push the gas pedal to the floor on your real passion and go all in on it. Pick one and go, and you will be infinitely more successful than if you try to do everything that seems to work for someone else.

Starting any new business or skill is going to be hard. It doesn't matter how easy it appears to be, there will always be more to it than meets the eye. But nothing is impossible. Find what you truly love to do and chase after it. Don't let anyone or anything deter you from it. This life is yours, and you need to do with it what you feel is right for YOU. Do that, and I promise you will be successful.

## The Cornerstone of Success: Habits

At the heart of consistency lay habits. These routines, seemingly mundane, shape our days and, in reality, our lives. My commitment to fitness wasn't an overnight decision, but rather a habit I cultivated over the years. Regular exercise, adequate sleep, and a balanced diet became cornerstones of my life. I knew the benefits of implementing them consistently, and the detriments of not doing so. I knew that if I wanted to live the life I desired, these had to become non-negotiables. And in doing so, they shaped my life in ways greater than I even imagined.

In 1997, when I was shot, I believe that my history of living a healthy lifestyle and staying in shape played a big role in my recovery. A strong foundation in a house or building can withstand the worst types of storms. As such, our bodies, when taken care of and treated with respect, can rebound from unimaginable adversities. If I hadn't made my body healthy and tough with my habits, I'm not sure I would still be here today.

If you haven't heard of James Clear, he's the author of the book called *Atomic Habits*. It's a fantastic read on how influential any and all types of habits can change your entire life. There are easy strategies to help you form better habits and kick the bad ones. But in the book, Clear talks about setting the goal to get 1% better every day. It seems like a small thing, but that singular focus of trying to be better by 1% every single day has immense consequences. On the other hand, the result of getting 1% worse every day might shock you. The book dives into the mechanics of habits, the ripple effects they can have, and the consistent changes that will ensue as a result of these habits. So, this 1% idea, let's do the math of how significant this can really be:

1% improvement every day for a year:

$$1.01^{365} = 37.8, \text{ or about 37x better.}$$

1% worse every day for a year:

$$99^{365} = .03, \text{ or 97\% decline.}$$

So, you can either get 37x better within a year, or take your skills and abilities almost completely down to zero. Those are vastly different. And this improvement or loss can be applied to just about any skill, from personal training to being a writer, painter, musician. The math above highlights the significant influence habits can have on your life. Habits will literally make or break us and are the silent architects of our destiny.

If you're wondering how to even start getting to that point, James Clear talks about the practice of "habit stacking."

That's where you stack one new habit on top of an already existing one. For example, right after you eat dinner, go on a ten-minute walk. You're going to eat, anyway, so start by adding new habits on top of unavoidable ones. Don't go crazy. Add one habit to your routine and try to stay consistent with it every day for at least a month. Then, if you think you're ready to add another, do so. Try to hit that one five to seven days per week consistently, but working your way to seven days a week should be the goal. It can be daunting to try to change your whole routine all at once. Start small, make it easy for you, and go from there. Rome wasn't built in a day, and neither was "The Rock."

As you navigate your way through your journey of life, remember this: it's not always about the grand gestures or monumental shifts in one's routine, or some great discovery. More often than not, it's about showing up day in and day out and putting in the work. Even if you love it, you have to work. Those tiny, seemingly insignificant habits, over time, sculpt your future for better or for worse.

## **Takeaways**

1. **Prioritize consistent, daily action over intensity.**
   Consistency doesn't have to mean taking huge leaps. Start with small steps that you know you can do on a regular basis. Whether it's related to fitness, business,

or personal growth, focus on regularity over the size of your efforts. Eventually, you start to build a discipline and that regularity becomes molded into your non-negotiable routine.

2. **Establish your key habits.** Make a list of your key habits that can be implemented into your daily regimen. Discover the habits that can act as the pillars for your own well-being and success. Take your key habits, try to add them to your already existing non-negotiables, and stack a new one right up against an old one.

3. **Embrace the 1% improvement rule.** Instead of trying to make massive changes overnight, make the effort to get just 1% better every day. Over time, these small increments can compound significantly and lead to some serious growth. On the other hand, a 1% decline daily can completely wipe you out in the long run. So, focus on daily improvements, no matter how minor they seem.

# Chapter 5

# The Importance of Routine and Balance

*"We are what we repeatedly do. Excellence, then, is not an act, but a habit."*

**Aristotle, philosopher**

Routine and balance, two words that might seem lackadaisical or in the "Yeah, I know" category. However, they can become two prime ingredients in the secret sauce to not just your business success, but to your overall personal well-being, as well. From seeing my dad with his routines and balance with his business, to coming over to America, I realized that my routines have been my anchor during times of uncertainty.

Life can get pretty crazy and messy at times. It's inevitable. What Matthew McConaughey would consider yellow or red lights in life. But routines and maintaining the best balance possible can help keep you upright during these times.

So many people get overwhelmed and feel trapped when life throws a touch of crazy at them. When you're grounded in routines and habits, and you know the list of non-negotiables, it provides you with a sense of direction. Having such things in place gives you enough direction to keep each day on track the best you can, and the rest can be filled in. You know where you have the time to put out certain fires and how you should go about each day, but don't sacrifice those non-negotiables. They might not seem profitable or advantageous in the short term, but they are what will help you be successful through this particular season of life.

## A Psychologist's Thoughts on Routine

Jordan Peterson is a world-renowned Canadian psychologist and thinker. He has often spoken about the power of routine and habits, emphasizing that they can keep an individual on track with their life goals. He suggests that

# JUST LIVE IT

setting up a schedule with daily and weekly routines and adhering to it as closely as possible offers structure, almost like a safety net, which holds people together during chaotic times. With where I've been and where I'm going, this message hit me pretty hard.

There's the old saying, "Idle hands are the devil's playground." And although not all who neglect a strict schedule are going to do heinous things, there is a good lesson behind the idea of being busy and in a routine. I have found that when my day is planned out, and I know what task needs to get done at a particular time, it is inherently more productive than when I try to go through my day by the seat of my pants. If I know I'm working on client plans from 9:00 a.m. to 1:00 p.m., then I have lunch from 1:00 p.m. to 2:00 p.m., then I'm working out from 3:00 p.m. to 4:30 p.m., there are a number of benefits. This is just a hypothetical schedule, but you get the idea.

But with this type of routine, I stay on task, and I stay focused during those times. I know I only have a certain amount of time to complete those particular objectives for that day, and so there are fewer distractions. There's no screwing around because the things *have* to get done. You'd also be amazed how much you can get done when you silence the notifications on your phone.

Initially coming to America, it was overwhelming, scary, and made me unsure of myself. Then add in being poor, jumping from city to city, living in my car, working odd jobs to barely make ends meet, and it was a rough start to a new life. But what kept me grounded were the things that I *was* certain of (bear in mind, some of these I did the best I could until I had better resources and conditions): quality sleep, proper nutrition, and regular exercise. Sure, I had to get creative with these for a while, but it was the act of having some consistency to my routine. They were things I knew, was familiar and comfortable with, and honestly kept me sane. I wasn't about to give up after a few hardships. The simple act of waking up at the same time, dedicating specific hours to training, and eating regular meals gave me a sense of control, even when so many things around me were uncertain.

## The Simplifying Life to Maintain Energy Balance

Now, routine doesn't mean cramming every minute of your day with activities. It's also about understanding where to channel your energies to maintain a balance. Over the years, especially in my entrepreneurial journey, I learned the importance of decluttering. This wasn't just about physical possessions but also about commitments, relationships, and goals.

In the midst of my professional bodybuilding pursuits, I ventured into several businesses. Trying to make it within that community is expensive. The food, supplements, entering shows, traveling to those shows, hotels, it all adds up. Coming from a war-torn country, I obviously didn't have much when I landed in the States. That's why I started working as hard as I could—I didn't want to stay at the bottom. I knew I could do better for myself, but I also knew it was all up to me. So, the allure of multitasking and diversifying was strong. But there were days I felt drained, spread too thin across my commitments.

After some time, I realized the necessity to simplify every new business I wanted in on. We talked earlier about the pitfalls of "shiny object syndrome" and how much that can hinder your progress. Fortunately, I was successful in my ventures, but I knew I had to narrow my focus. When I just focused on fixing and flipping cars, I ended up with my own car lot. When the focus was cell phones, the business boomed (before being undercut, of course). And after turning pro and the fitness business started rolling, I knew that was *the* thing that I needed to keep my eyes on. No more distractions, no more fast-money hustles. My vision was to help people with health and fitness, and now that I was there, I needed to stick to that vision.

Keeping this focus on what truly mattered, and which brought joy meant sometimes saying "no" to friends or fun things. It meant prioritizing other tasks and aligning everything with my core values and mission. This conscious prioritizing and decluttering helped me maintain my energy balance, ensuring I didn't burn out.

Many times, you'll see not just entrepreneurs, but especially entrepreneurs, experience burnout. It can usually be as a result of a few things: not truly passionate about the thing they're working on, spreading themselves too thin, not right with themselves, doing too much and not hiring to accommodate workload. Energy is the fuel for the engine, and you can't operate on "empty" forever. I had to become more selfish with my time and focus.

It's a common theme for entrepreneurs to start to really minimize their circle and be more selective with the things they go do and say "yes" to. It's not because we don't like our friends, but we're on missions that are higher than ourselves. And to maintain this steady stream of energy and to avoid burnout the best you can, you have to have a solid core of systems and healthy habits.

## The Significance of Rest, Sleep, and Understanding One's Energy Rhythms

Clearly, I'm a big advocate of physical fitness and overall wellness. But I think this still gets undervalued in how intertwined those things are with our mental and emotional states, as well.

# JUST LIVE IT

One aspect that rings true across entrepreneurship and bodybuilding is pushing your body to its limits. And in both worlds, it's not just celebrated but almost looked down upon if you don't subscribe to this mantra.

Early on, I learned the value of sleep. Especially after I had been shot, my body needed to rest and recover. It's how the body can recover from quite literally almost everything. There's no time I can think of when your body being under-slept is advantageous. My body was strong due to years of training and proper nutrition, but its recovery, to a great extent, was supported by quality rest and understanding my energy rhythms. That is when I do my best work and training throughout the day.

Every person has a unique energy cycle; times when they are most productive and times when they need to wind down. For example, some people love to work out early in the morning before the sun is even up, and others do better later in the day. Personally, I like to get my body moving and have some morning routines we'll get into in the next chapter, but I don't go train right away. I like to get things started, see how everything is feeling, set my body up best for the day, and go from there. With work, there are those who are most creative as soon as they wake up, and those who are night owls who are most productive into the later hours.

I have one friend who is both. He is super sharp mentally in the mornings, slower in the afternoons, and ramps up again from dinnertime until the early morning hours of the next day. Me being me, I had to tell him, "Dude! You have to pick one because you have to sleep!" He then told me, "Don't worry; I get my six hours." I just shook my head and told him that's not sustainable. We all need at least seven to eight hours of sleep each night.

Matthew Walker is a British scientist and neuroscience professor at the University of California, Berkeley. One of his main areas of study is sleep, lack thereof, and how both can affect the human body. It's actually quite scary how detrimental poor sleep can have on us. And there are people who go years with poor sleep quality, going through life tired and run down. Walker was on the Joe Rogan podcast once, and he mentioned this idea that people say they can operate on six hours of sleep. He continued to claim that few people in the world can actually function at optimal levels on six hours of sleep. Very few people in the *world*.

So, if you think you're one of these outliers, it's highly unlikely. And if you're reading this, thinking about your bad sleeping habits, there are a few things you can do to start improving your sleep today:

- Set a bedtime and stick to it every night.
- Stop eating ninety to a hundred twenty minutes before bedtime.

# JUST LIVE IT

- Your room should be cool (but don't freeze yourself) and dark.
- Try to cut off screens thirty to sixty minutes before bedtime.
- Try to limit bright lights/exposure to lights thirty minutes before bedtime.
- When you first wake up, don't let the first thing you do be looking at your phone screen and starting to scroll through social media, emails, and texts. Turn the alarm off and start getting up.

Your sleep is *the* most important part of your regimen, first only to proper nutrition. The thing is, you can skip a meal, if it gets to be too late at night. If you just had a long day and aren't able to eat dinner, that's much less detrimental than getting poor sleep. Now, I understand if you're starving late at night because you didn't get time to eat much at all. You could either drink some water to try to curb cravings, but if you're so hungry that you won't fall asleep, then you could try something light:

- A couple egg whites.
- A couple handfuls of mixed nuts.
- Veggies and hummus.
- Some fruit.

You want to keep it light because you're about to go to sleep. Don't try to be comfortably full, or full much at all. Ideally, you'd go to sleep, but I know life happens.

Life, especially in the modern rat race society, can often feel like a juggling act. And I never learned how to juggle! It's not about how many balls you can keep in the air, but rather about mastering the art of balance. Now, that doesn't mean you keep adding as much as humanly possible after you feel like you've achieved a little balance with the balls already in the air. You must maintain the balance.

Back to our idea of saying "no" to more things. That's a skill that you need to work on in order to block out unnecessary distractions and noises. Because when you finally start hitting your stride and doing what you believe you're called to do in this life, then you will be met with even more resistance. From shiny object syndrome to people not wanting you to do better than them, things and people will try to get in your way. No matter what, stay laser focused on your goals and vision. Establishing a routine will help maintain that tunnel vision. Routines and habits help simplify life, and understanding your energy rhythms are more than just strategies; they are lifelines that have anchored me throughout my journey. I share this in the hope that they provide guidance, comfort, and a roadmap for you as you navigate your own unique journey of life. Remember, life is a marathon, not a sprint. Embrace it with routine and balance.

## Takeaways

1. **Establish a morning routine.** Begin your day with intention. Whether it's a quick workout, a meditation session, or simply reading for fifteen minutes or a certain number of pages, create some sort of routine that sets the tone for the day ahead. Consistent morning actions ground you, provide clarity on what has to happen throughout any given day, and offer a sense of accomplishment before the day's chaos gets rolling. Even on the most unpredictable days, a solid morning routine becomes your anchor, offering familiarity, stability, and a sense of having control of your life.

2. **Prioritize and declutter your commitments.** Take a step back and evaluate your commitments that crowd your daily, weekly, and monthly life. Also recognize the things that tend to come up last minute. Are they aligned with your goals and values? Are the people around you helping or hurting your progress toward those goals and values? Sometimes, you have to make cuts and having less is more. With less noise and clutter, you have more time to accomplish the important tasks, more room to breathe, and more space to create the life you want. Saying "no" isn't a sign of weakness, quite the opposite in fact. Being able to say "no" is a

testament to your dedication to yourself, your goals, and the value you have of your self-worth and time.

3. **Recognize your energy peaks.** When do you tend to get the most done? Do you have certain projects that you like to do at certain times in the day? Instead of fighting against your natural rhythm, lean into it. Pick out those most ideal times for particular projects and use that high energy and focus to knock out the biggest, hardest tasks. And conversely, during your energy lulls, engage in lighter, more mindless tasks that don't require as much energy and effort. This level of self-awareness helps you optimize productivity while making sure you're not spreading yourself too thin or draining yourself, thus leading to burnout.

# Chapter 6

# Following The Natural Way

*"Let food be thy medicine and medicine be they food."*

**Hippocrates, philosopher**

Few things have the power to shape us more profoundly than our habits and choices, especially when it comes to health and wellness. As we make our way through this chapter, we'll dive deep into the essence of following nature's path and doing things the more natural way. Think of it almost as a guidebook etched into our very beings. We'll explore the importance of nourishing our bodies with the right foods, embracing a lifestyle that radiates balance, and understanding the spiritual benefits that come from aligning with our true selves.

My personal journey, full of ups and downs, has given me insights that I hope will shed light on these topics. They helped save my life, and the lives of others. Now, hopefully, they can help many more. Remember that our lives are a testament to our choices, and by opting for the natural way, we can carve out a life filled with purpose, authenticity, and a long life of good health and blessings.

## A Battle Against Time and Disease

On August 13th, 2017, exactly twenty years to the day that I was shot, I faced another evil foe that would become one of the greatest challenges of my life—cancer. That word itself scares anyone who hears it. At first, I started having a hard time peeing. So, I saw a urologist first, and they brushed it off as no big thing and prescribed me something to help. But then I started to not feel good and was having some stomach pains, preventing me from going to the bathroom at all. I saw a colorectal surgeon before leaving town for a speaking engagement, and he also brushed it off as no big deal. He thought it was just hemorrhoids, but it kept getting worse. I still went on the trip, and by the time I had gotten to Italy, I was in agony. It was so painful that I could hardly function and was still unable to go to the bathroom in any capacity.

# JUST LIVE IT

The lady I was doing the seminar for told me that her husband was a colon doctor, so I told him of my symptoms, and he gave me something to go to the bathroom. Then he performed an endoscopy. The doctor told me I had 90% blockage and had a lot of cancer inside of me. It was stage 3c colorectal cancer.

After having studied Dr. Goswami with Quantum University, he talked extensively about the alkaline diet, which is based on the theory that a lot of the foods we eat can cause our bodies to produce excess acid, leading to a lot of different health issues. During my bodybuilding days, and during the career of almost every bodybuilder, we eat a ton of different animal meats and proteins, and it's not all perfect. But the shear quantities we eat definitely doesn't help the cause. The alkaline diet, however, is basically a plant-based diet, containing mostly vegetables, fruits, whole grains, beans/lentils, nuts, seeds, and no alcohol. So, when I found out about my cancer and got back to Rochester, I saw another doctor and changed my diet immediately to the alkaline diet, keeping it mostly raw vegan.

They immediately got me into surgery to start removing the cancer, but they didn't know how much it had spread. Because of that, they ended up taking out my bladder and prostate. As a result, I now have an ostomy bag for the rest of my life. For those who don't know what that is, it's a bag that is attached to my abdomen surgically so that bodily waste can flow freely into the bag. I empty it when I need to, and that's how I go to the bathroom. In total, I went through thirteen different surgeries.

I'll tell you one thing; I'd give all the money I have to go back to my pre-cancer health. Knowing then what I know now would've saved me from all of this. But you know me, turn every negative into a positive.

With everything that was going on, I still tried my best to hang on to that notion. In fact, I was in such good spirits that I was still coaching people while I was in the hospital. Clients of mine were training to go to the Olympia, and they weren't going to quit on me, so I wasn't going to quit on them. That, coupled with the fact that I absolutely love what I do, there was no way I wasn't seeing it through to the end with my people. And you know what? They made it to Olympia!

Even though times seemed dark, there was no way that this was the end of my story. God sent me back before, and if it were my time, I wouldn't be healing as I was. He didn't need me yet, because other people did.

My journey through chemo treatment was one of the most revealing eye-openers I've ever witnessed. With disbelief, the other patients getting their chemo in the same room as me were being fed (in my opinion) the very foods that probably helped lead to them getting sick in the first place. They were all getting unhealthy foods, like pizza, bologna sandwiches, and candy while receiving their chemo

# JUST LIVE IT

treatments. This is the exact problem! They're fed this silly food pyramid that was arbitrarily made up from the food industry, then given these harsh drugs to help fight the diseases that same food pyramid helped give them. Then they are fed the same foods again during those treatments.

Firsthand, I saw the vicious cycle that so many people go through, particularly here in America. I'm not trying to bash America, only their food system and food industry. How many overweight Europeans do you see?

Through all of my treatments, I was the only one who didn't lose his hair, never got nauseous, and I was still working out. As a matter of fact, instead of losing a bunch of weight, like most cancer patients do, I was gaining it! My energy was fantastic, and I breezed through my chemo treatments. How many people can say that? I dare you to find me ten.

After five5onths of my treatment and new diet, my CA-125 levels (a reading that indicates the likelihood of someone having cancer) was at now 0. The normal range is between 0 and 35 U/ml. After five months, I was at 0. The more naturally I ate, the faster I healed.

They had also put me on a bunch of opioids, another rabbit hole I can easily go down. Look, I'm one of the happiest guys on the planet, but these opioid drugs made me have a lot of dark, suicidal thoughts. It got so bad that I didn't remember seeing my family over the holidays because the painkillers had put me in such a daze. It was scary that I couldn't recall moments like those and made me sad that I lost those memories. But those drugs paired with the poor diets here, it's no wonder how many people are sick and riddled with all the different diseases.

I started using gummies with THC & CBD and was able to get off every single opioid in about six to seven weeks. So, to those skeptical about using alternative options, like THC & CBD, they work. Since starting them, I never had any more suicidal thoughts. It's much better on my system as a whole and helped me a lot more than those drugs ever would.

There's a documentary called *Weed the People.* It covers the effects that such compounds from the cannabis plant can have on various diseases. Within the documentary, they showed a petri dish with both cancer cells, and then THC & CBD cannabinoids. All of a sudden, the THC was basically eating the cancer cells. The THC looked like little worms and the cancer cells were these black spots. The little worms would move closer to the cancer cells and just suck it up, and it was gone. It was literally *eating* the cancer. I'm not saying it's a cure for cancer, but I'm saying it helped me and has been shown to help others. And the THC was often administered in high concentrations, via edible or IV. They weren't smoking it and getting high; it was truly used for medicinal purposes. And it worked. But, in my case, I used the gummies to get off the pain meds. But again, it worked.

# JUST LIVE IT

Through my battle, the more I adhered to natural foods, the faster my body responded. Unlike many going through the same treatments, I felt exactly as a cancer patient shouldn't. How does that grab ya? But the path still wasn't without its challenges.

The pain and mental torment from all the surgeries and medications I'd already taken were pretty unbearable at times. Drawing from my own spiritual beliefs, as well as teachings from Dr. Lipton and Dr. Dispenza, I understood the power of the mind and spirit in healing. The belief that our body, like a house, can be fixed and rebuilt. All of these factors played a major role in my recovery.

With how well I did with a serious cancer, doctors were reaching out and asking me what I was doing. When I would tell them, they would be absolutely blown away. They couldn't believe how much I was able to heal myself with diet, and that part made me sad. All those years of medical school with some of the most brilliant people, and they simply aren't taught (in-depth) the one thing that can have the biggest impact on anything and everything else.

As time passed and word spread, patients started to reach out to me, asking for help, and I even had another doctor hand a patient of his off to me who was diagnosed with terminal cancer.

In 2019, about the time I was completely cancer free, a doctor told me about this patient that he was performing surgery on in a few days, to remove as much as he could. "Hey, doc, after you're done, get her in touch with me and send her my way," I said to him. He reinforced the fact that she had cancer all over her body and was going to die. "That's fine," I said. "Do your surgery and send her to me, anyway." Reluctantly, he took my information.

I wasn't sure if he'd actually send her my way, but sure enough, she reached out a couple weeks later. I managed her diet completely, and in 2020, she was cancer free. One year is all it took working with me for her cancer to be completely gone.

Another gentleman had found me over the internet, and he needed a kidney transplant. I took over his entire nutrition plan, and one of the biggest things I removed was fish. After some time, his biomarkers improved to where he no longer needed the transplant.

You might find a few studies and articles on diet therapy or how some foods may help prevent cancer. But you won't find any claiming to be able to cure cancer with food. I won't speak to the intentions of healthcare workers, but I'm not sure how many are supposed to figure out and know what I figured out and know: your food can kill you or heal you. The doctors wanted me to go on dialysis, but since being on my alkaline and vegan diet, there's no need for that anymore. If I had held off on the surgery where they removed my bladder and prostate, there is no question that I could have prevented them from removing either, just by fixing my diet sooner.

When something is going wrong with your body, or something seems off, that's your body telling you that something is wrong or off. Don't ignore it, thinking it'll pass or get better on its own. It's possible, but you have to help it help itself. Our bodies were so brilliantly and beautifully made by God. We are meant to be able to heal. If the body can't do so, then it's your job to figure out why. What is preventing it from getting better? It's not a lack of medications; I know that much.

Throughout this ordeal, I encountered numerous testimonies of the healing power of food and mindset. I worked with individuals who, through dietary changes and mental resilience, reversed dire diagnoses and regained their health. Don't tell me food can't cure people and diseases. And don't believe anyone who says it's not possible. I, and others I've coached, are living proof of it.

In a later chapter, I will go through some daily hacks, if you will, and health and wellness tips that I think can be done by and good for the masses.

## Staying Ture and Honest: The Spiritual Beliefs

During my pursuit of health and wellness, I've learned that your physical well-being is deeply connected to your spiritual well-being. Staying true to oneself, always telling the truth, and living authentically can resonate at a deeper level. But at the core of it all needs to be a belief in a higher power.

I'm a strong believer in God. I recently watched a video of an agnostic man ask a theologian to not prove that God is real, but that there is a reason to be on the side that it is more likely that God created everything over the Big Bang. The theologian thanked him for his genuine question and dove right in.

To keep track, we'll call the theologian Simon and the agnostic Paul. So, Simon starts every presentation of his case in a similar fashion: "In my personal experience in life ..." and then will continue further. At the crux of it all, Simon kept coming back to the same conclusion, and that is that he has only seen life come from life. If you think about it, what thing that contains life and is truly living, ever came from something that is not? A human does not come from a machine without life. No, it comes from another human with life. Same with animals. As a result, the idea that a clashing of rocks and planets created lifeforms that would eventually evolve into humans is much harder to lean on than that something with life created a universe of more life. I was blown away.

It seems simple, but that argument alone cannot be disproven. This is not the argument to prove that God is real; it was merely presented as a way to try to convince someone that God is the more likely option than the Big Bang Theory.

# JUST LIVE IT

Before anyone starts calling me, yelling about this argument, remember that I'm just the one sharing the information! But it does make you think ...

Spirituality, my unwavering belief in God has been a guiding force. It not only offers solace during the toughest of times but also grants clarity and purpose to life's journey. Without God, I wouldn't still be here. It's amazing the divine plan that He has. It's not up to us. We control what we can, but ultimately, it all comes down to God's planning. As painful as some parts may be, as awful as getting shot and cancer was, the inconveniences they've each left me with is God's plan is nothing short of perfect. It is through His gifting of talents and life that we're all able to do amazing things.

We get one shot at this life, so we must take care of ourselves, each other, and make this world a better place than how we found it. We're on borrowed time, so we should live a life worth living that emulates how we were made and meant to live: in His image and likeness.

Within the past year, there have been countless athletes speaking out more about their faith than any other time I can remember. And not just sports, but famous Hollywood celebrities, too. We live in a satanic culture where the only things sought after are pleasures. No longer do we seem to actually fear God, and it shows. Our entire world is acting a fool, like nothing bad is happening or will happen, and if our society keeps going on like that, we're eventually going to be in for a rude awakening, in this life or the next.

## The Power of Mindset and Purpose

I've mentioned I take every negative and turn it into a positive. When you couple that mindset with the idea that everything happens *for* us rather than *to* us, we're able to take on a whole different outlook. Every challenge, every setback, is an opportunity to grow and learn. When we embrace this notion, we see adversities as fuel, propelling us forward instead of weighing us down. It also forces us to take a sense of ownership and personal responsibility.

I remember a friend of mine, years ago, said during one hard season of his life, he would call his mom and just start ranting. He wasn't too happy with his day job, the girlfriend he had, or really anything going on in his life. He'll even admit to this day that he had everything. Now, he wasn't loaded by any means, but to a lot of people, he had everything. But he lost his purpose and fell into the "woe is me" mindset. So, he'd call his mom, barely saying hello, if at all, and he'd just start going on about how terrible everything was going. Being the great mom she is, she'd listen and talk him off the ledge, calming him down to change his outlook and move on to live another day. To this day, I'm not sure how that kind of stress didn't make him drop dead some moments!

# JUST LIVE IT

Outside of a lot of different factors, he followed up by saying that his mom told him something that not only changed his mindset on a dime, but it's something he promised to carry with him forever and share with those who were ready for it.

During one of his infamous rants to his mom on the telephone, she told him that he is exactly where he is in his life because of every single decision he ever made. Nobody else.

Let me say that again. We are all in the very place we are in because of every decision we have ever made.

Mark today, as you read that line again, as the last day you live in any sort of victim mindset ever again. It's done.

I've been shot three times and had thirteen surgeries to remove stage 3 cancer. I wasn't a victim then, and I'm not going to be a victim now. The faster we all take responsibility for ourselves and realize it's our own decision-making that got us in the situations we complain about, the faster those decisions start to change.

Andy Frisella, CEO of the supplement company 1st Phorm, was on a podcast and harping on this very idea about victimhood. Within his rant, he says, "The only noble thing about victimhood is overcoming it."

It's never too late to take back control of your life, but there might be some painful acceptances that need to come before you do. You also have to make sure you're fulfilling what you believe to be your purpose.

One metric I like to put up against what someone does for their work every day is this: if you wake up on the wrong side of the bed and just don't want to deal with it that day, what is the one type of work you'd still actually kind of enjoy going to do when you're in a bad mood?

Even with the best dream job in the world, there will still be days when it feels like work, but those days can feel pretty all right. But your mindset and purpose have to be right.

When this shift starts to happen, and you consciously see the changes take place and how you evolve, it becomes addicting. It's impossible to go back to your old ways. You see everything so differently and get to undergo massive changes. You may outgrow certain friends and start to chase more grandiose dreams that are much bigger than yourself. Purpose and mindset. When they start to align, you become dangerous. Welcome to the other side.

## **Takeaways**

1. **Prioritize natural nutrition.** Begin by assessing your diet. Are you consuming processed foods that are high in sugar and unhealthy fats? Start by slowly incorporating more whole foods into your daily meals. Opt for multicolored fruits and vegetables, whole grains, and lean proteins. Remember, the food we consume is the fuel our body runs on. Give your body

premium fuel, and you'll witness profound changes in energy, mood, and overall well-being.

2. **Spiritual alignment.** Spend a few moments each day in introspection. Whether it's through prayer, meditation, or simply quiet reflection, connect with your inner self and the greater universe. This spiritual grounding not only enhances your mental clarity and emotional stability but also keeps you true to your life's purpose.

3. **Listen to your body.** Your body often sends signals when something's off. Whether it's fatigue, constant headaches, or digestive issues, take them as cues. Instead of seeking a quick fix, dig deeper to find the root cause. Often, a change in diet, mindset, or daily routine can alleviate these symptoms. Remember the story of my battle against cancer and the vital role my dietary and lifestyle changes played? Your body is an incredible machine; treat it with care and respect.

# Chapter 7

# Measurement, Management, and Enjoying the Journey

*"How wonderful it is that nobody need wait a single moment before starting to improve the world."*

**Anne Frank, Jewish diarist during Nazi Germany**

    Throughout my career, both as an entrepreneur and as a bodybuilder, I've measured *a lot*. I've measured thousands of meals and what their macro breakdowns were (macros are proteins, carbs, and fats), countless workouts and weight progressions, revenues and costs for multiple businesses, biomarkers for cancer—you name it, I've measured and tracked it, for myself and for others. There's a great saying that, "What gets measured, gets managed." In my journey, this principle has held true every step of the way. Measuring is not just for the sake of recording. Yes, it's important to know where your numbers are at, in all these areas, at all times. But when you measure, you're able to understand, adapt, and grow at a much more efficient rate than if you weren't. If you're not measuring, then you don't care. Think about it. If you're running a business and you have no idea how much money is going out, what it's being spent on, have no clue what's coming in and where it's being allocated, then you're clueless. You have to measure and manage your business, so you know where it is and where it needs to go.

The same is true for bodybuilders. If you don't know the amount of food you're eating, the macro and caloric breakdown, then you're just flying blind, throwing shit at the wall and hoping something sticks. Think about something that you keep track of in your daily life. Odds are high that you care a whole lot about that thing. If you're not tracking, you do not care enough to progress in that thing. Because what gets measured, gets managed.

# GEORGE FARAH, PHD

# The Art of Measuring Progress

Tracking food and weight is a pain. There's no two ways about it. Some clients love it because they need that strict guidance and accountability, and with others, it stresses them out, and they want me to tell them what to eat and exactly how much of it to eat every day. That's fine, as long as they stick to it. But it's all about the power of data and context.

The more data you have, the more informed decisions you can make. You can even measure your personal life. What do you think is missing, if anything, at the current moment? Now, how has that area of your life gone in the past? What has led you to this exact moment? What are some constants you've noticed when things go extremely well versus when they don't?

It's easy to feel lost without benchmarks. You have no direction, and you fly blind, hoping things just magically work out. They might, but it's unlikely.

When you set a goal or specific number, now you have something to aim for. You know where you're heading, now you just have to engineer the plan to get you there.

Like setting milestones for personal and professional achievements, the weight room taught me the importance of setting, measuring, and adjusting goals. It taught me that success isn't about reaching a final destination, but about understanding and appreciating every step of the way. But if you want to make real progress, you have to measure and manage your progress.

## Embracing the Process, Especially When It's Hard

You have to love it. One might argue you have to be obsessed with it. We talked before about being obsessed with the beautiful grind. It's not always going to be the most fun thing ever. Even your passions require you to "work." But when it gets hard, you have to remember why you started, and you must hang on to that in moments that test you more than you think you can handle it. The ones who hang on are the ones who make it.

There's a unique thrill in lifting heavier weights, setting new personal records, feeling the struggle of that last rep, and locking it out. I recently had a client who we pushed her weights in a strict shoulder press with dumbbells. She looked at me like I was crazy. I mean, maybe a little bit, but hey, we all need some of that! I told her she could do it. I had a rep range in my head, but I didn't share it with her, because this was about feeling that hard struggle under the weight and pushing through it. When I saw the struggle I was looking for and saw her fighting through it, I told her, "One more." She fought through that last one then set them down. She looked at me with a, "Whew." She was tired, and I was grinning from ear-to-ear. "That's what I'm talking about!" She caught her breath, and I explained to her why we did what we had just done. Our next set, we took it back down five pounds, but she felt the struggle and pushed forward. She embraced it, knowing it was going to be heavy, knowing it was going to be hard, and went through the fire, anyway.

During my time in the hospital, I still found joy in coaching others. Even from that cold, fluorescent-lit room, I was preparing folks for Olympia because they still had the fight in them, and so did I. I loved what I was doing. I was obsessed. Coaching was my passion, a lifeline. The more I gave to the sport and its athletes, the more strength I drew from it. It became evident that if you truly love what you do, you'll find a way to keep doing it, no matter the odds.

## Prioritizing Self-Care: The Oxygen Mask Analogy

I've flown thousands of miles and hundreds of times. Not sure the last time I actually paid 100% attention to the safety announcements (oops), but one day, I was just watching, and it hit me when they talked about if the oxygen masks drop down. "Put on your oxygen mask before assisting others." I finally realized the depth of those words.

Even though I was in the hospital while coaching, I was still prioritizing my own well-being way before then. Even then,

*I* was the priority. But if I were going to have to lay there anyway while taking care of myself, I might as well help take care of others if I could.

No matter how invincible we might feel, there will be moments when our body and mind yell for some attention. Don't ignore those. Your body is trying to tell you something. While I've pushed a lot of boundaries with my body, I never lost sight of the importance of self-care.

Taking care of and prioritizing yourself isn't selfish; it's necessary. Never feel bad for taking care of you first.

When I was sound mentally, physically, and spiritually, I was able to give more to those around me. They got my best self because I worked on becoming my best self. It's a simple yet glaring truth: you cannot pour from an empty cup. You need to fill your cup up daily, however that looks for you. Feed your body with nourishing foods, challenge it with hard workouts, recharge it with quality sleep, and reinforce it with positive thoughts and affirmations.

## **Takeaways**

1. **Embrace quantifiable progress.** It's essential to track your progress in all things. Setting clear, measurable goals provides direction and motivation. Whether it's in your career, fitness, or personal life, take time to

regularly review your achievements and adjust your approach based on what the numbers tell you.

2. **Find passion in the process.** Challenges are inevitable, but when you're passionate about something, even hard obstacles become manageable. Enjoy every step in your journey, because it all molds you into the person you hope to become. You'll learn to enjoy the ride along the way rather than the finish line.

3. **Prioritize your well-being.** Like the oxygen mask analogy, you need to put yourself first. You can't pour from an empty cup and give it to others when you're running on empty. Taking care of yourself isn't selfish; it's necessary. By being at your best, you're better prepared to help those around you.

# Chapter 8

# Truth, Sacrifice, and the Lens of Clarity

*"How wonderful it is that nobody need wait a single moment before starting to improve the world."*

**Benjamin Franklin, Founding Father of the United States**

Sacrifices and clarity are necessary to get moving in the right direction for any venture. You need to know that you must give things up, say "no" more often than you ever have, and make your goals and mission abundantly clear so that you know which way to go. If you're willing to sacrifice for your dream and are clear on what that dream is, you're in a better spot to get moving in the right direction toward the end goal. The path to get there may change along the way, but the goal never should.

It also seems that, today, there is a lot of skewed information on what the real truth is, about anything. We live in an era dominated by the media and a slandering of those who disagree with us. Although we won't get super deep into politics, I do want to touch on similarities I've seen between the leadership of both Lebanon and America. Some may surprise you, some may not, and some may be harder to accept. But as someone who came from a country torn up by war, extremists, and interventions from all sorts of other countries that don't know our culture, I feel it is my duty to share my insights.

## Seeking Truth in a World of Deception

Our mindset isn't just for our own ventures, but to be able to think critically, logically, and rationally. All the happenings of the last few years, particularly this year with new wars, unhinged media, and society getting more divisive than I've seen in a long time, I felt compelled to touch upon it a little bit. Looking at my time spent in Lebanon and comparing it to the politics in America, the signs are eerily similar.

# JUST LIVE IT

The same people who ran Lebanon during the war are still in power, and things are looking grim again. It didn't seem that the government was for its people, but more so looking to strip them of as many rights as possible, tell them what was in their best interest, and retain power.

The news was not *for* or *by* the people, but a hand of the government showing how great of a job they were doing, when, in reality, things were getting increasingly worse.

What I see in America is all too similar to what I saw growing up and after moving to the States. Here, I see efforts to defend those who protect us because of a few bad apples. I see news that attacks political opponents on both sides, a society that lives to get emotional and irrational, and a loss of proud nationalism for one's country and beliefs. This government is a shame and is falling victim to the same broken system that I saw in the Middle East. The Nazis controlled the media, attacked political opponents, loved suppressing certain classes of people, didn't want citizens to bear arms, and were always ready for a war. Sound familiar? I'm speaking about these things because I have lived them once before, and I'm starting to live them again.

Our minds seek conflict and the urge to be the hero. And, in doing so, people often make things ten times worse. Nobody has been able to look me dead in the face and tell me things have gotten increasingly better over the years. We need to be free thinkers, have conversations with those we disagree with, be open-minded enough to be okay with having our minds changed, and accept when we're wrong. It's okay to be wrong, especially when you own it and move on to correct it. But we're not doing that. We doubled down.

When we get back to being proud of our country and each other, being okay with disagreement, and focus on helping ourselves before trying to police and help everyone else, we will be in a much better spot to help those who want and ask for it.

To wrap this up in a slightly lighter sense, I do think America is the greatest country in the world. What can't you do here? You can build any company you want and can grow it to be as big as you can imagine. If you spoke back to a cop in Lebanon, they might shoot you. Here, you can criticize your president without being sent to prison. We also reward people for doing things, like building and creating. Americans push people to be successful and be better. Other countries aren't known for doing things like that. You're here to be lifted up and do well. America is a beautiful place to live. Every country is going to have things it's trying to improve, but America has such freedoms and opportunities that half the world can only ever dream of.

# Takeaways

1. **Embrace self-accountability.** Much like the story of the client who used a past defeat as motivation, every setback can be viewed as an opportunity for growth. Instead of blaming external factors, taking responsibility allows you to identify areas of improvement, helping you become stronger and more resilient.
2. **Question the mainstream narrative.** No matter who it is, question everything. It's okay to ask questions, especially when the media is driving a not-so-hidden agenda. It's important to look at multiple sources and perspectives. Prioritize independent outlets, like podcasts and journalists without a special interest in money, which can provide the facts as they are presented and have unbiased reporting. Educate yourself and do your best to discern between agendas and the truth.
3. **Strive for personal excellence.** Inspired by the idea of impressing oneself, it's important to set personal goals. Continuously aim to surpass your own expectations. When you feel a deep satisfaction in your achievements, you'll know you're on the right path. Give yourself the chills. It's about the internal applause, not the external accolades.

# Chapter 9

# Living Life with Purpose

(The Pillars of Integrity and Consistency)

> *"The measure of who we are is what we do with what we have."*
>
> **Vince Lombardi, NFL coach**

We've talked about a few key characteristics that have helped me and others get on the path to becoming the best version of ourselves. From discipline to survival mode, there have been a few key elements. But two more things I need to add to the list are integrity and consistency. They have been foundational in every phase of my life. From being consistent with my own health and clients, to the integrity of being an honest man of servitude, a man whom I hope one day makes me proud of myself, but above all, someone who ultimately makes God proud.

## How You Do One Thing is How You Do Everything

You might have heard this one, but maybe not. When I first heard it, I had to think about it for a second. Was this true?

When I reminisced on all the people whom I have coached, and on my own life, I saw the consistencies. In the athlete world, they push themselves hard on the field, on stage, in the weight room, in a court. But you also see them pushing other areas of their lives. They might have a business that they're gung-ho about, or they're extremely involved in their family. They go hard in every aspect.

Think about if you're in school and have to type a paper. If you only put in a minimal effort, do you tend to work with the same intensity in other areas of your life?

I challenge you to check out your own consistency in how you do everything throughout your everyday life. Whether you have a small task, like tying your shoe, or have a big life decision to make, every action should be approached with equal dedication and purpose. Make the best decision you can on the trajectory of your life and do what's best for you. Tie the greatest knot those shoelaces have ever been tied into. Every action, no matter how small, is an opportunity to showcase your commitment to quality, precision, and your respect for the task at hand. I love this mantra. It keeps efforts consistent, as well as the outcomes.

## Significance of Self-Talk

How do you talk to yourself? What kind of thoughts do you put through your mind and into your body? They both can have a massive impact on your physique and life. I've experienced this, I've coached this—your thoughts and words to yourself can quite literally be the difference between you winning and losing.

Positive self-talk comes from having purpose, direction, and a strong idea of what you want out of this life. When you know what you want, have a long-term vision in place, and are mentally ready to attack, you can achieve greatness. But when the mind slips, or you hit a speed bump and start putting yourself down, it can affect everything and prevent the progress you're looking for.

I had this one guy come to me after he got beat pretty badly in a show. He signs with me, and I tell him to sign up for the exact same show for the following year. He was hesitant because, in his mind, he had been defeated. He was stressed out, unsure of what to do next, and came to me in distress.

Before we even talked about nutrition or training, we talked about mindset. I knew I could help this guy. The question was: could he help himself and get out of his own way? He didn't believe himself going into his last show, and his physique and results suffered as a result. So, I made sure he got right in the head, and then we got to work.

I told him he was going to win the next year, and once he believed it, everything changed. His training was more consistent and intense, he never missed a single meal, and he did all the extra work he could in a day. He felt the hunger again.

So, we go to the same show that he had lost, and he straight up tells the other guys, "I don't know what you're all doing here. I'm here to win." It's like he took a page out of my book when I handed the judges my business card! Man, I was so proud of his confidence! And he mopped the floor with his competition. I mean, it wasn't even a question that he was the clear winner. Then he went on to the New York Pro show and won that, as well. In a year's time, he was ready to quit and didn't think he had it anymore, to become a professional bodybuilder.

The body will follow the mind in either direction. Your thoughts and self-talk are extremely important. If you've ever read *The Hidden Messages in Water*, you'll know where I'm going with this.

Our bodies are 60% water, and that book studies the effects that positive and negative energy can have on water. The same is true for humans. When we're all pent up, full of negative emotion and energy, everything feels worse in our entire body. But when you start to be nicer to yourself, look more positively at things, and try to put out positive energy, you can turn your entire mood around in seconds. So, the next time something isn't going right, or maybe you're prepping for a bodybuilding show, always remember the impact that positive self-talk can have.

## Integrity and Consistent Character

I was listening to a podcast where the host was talking about the idea of wearing multiple hats. It's the notion that you should act a certain way in this environment or that environment, talk a different way to certain people. And I get where people might tailor their communication style for various reasons, but the podcast host actually spoke pretty strongly against this. In his delivery, the rationale behind not being a supporter of wearing multiple hats was that he believes in being the same guy to everyone, being consistent so people knew what they were going to get. But also, it was his way of staying true to his character. Why should he have

# JUST LIVE IT

to alter himself for people? Not that he was being outwardly mean or rude, but he spoke the same to the guest on the show as he would his wife, as he would to his friends. It was full of respect, humility, a genuine curiosity, but he was also strong in his beliefs. He stood his ground.

After thinking about it, I don't think I changed myself for anybody. I'm a happy guy who loves training, business, and helping other people as much as possible. I turn negatives into positives and try to live life as a man of God. My goal is to always live that way and be consistent with it.

The other benefit of living as yourself all the time is that people know who and what they're going to get. Imagine always being a rollercoaster of reactions and emotions, making people have no idea the type of version of you that they're about to get. I'm not sure that's the healthiest thing for anyone, so there might be something else going on there. But when you can be your genuine self even 90% of the time, I think you'll find a lot more happiness in your daily life by just sticking to who and what you are. It's a pretty free way to live.

Living with consistent integrity and positive self-talk is hard. Some days, everything just goes sideways. It's okay to have an off day, but I'd encourage you to find a healthy outlet on those days to get yourself back to equilibrium.

In embracing these principles, I've not only found success in my professional journey but have discovered an incredible sense of inner peace. I hope you try to embrace some of these values, because they can offer an abundant and happy life. And that's what I want for everyone. How you do anything is how you do everything. So, choose wisely and make every action count.

# **Takeaways**

1. **Mindful execution.** Try to incorporate the mantra of "how you do anything is how you do everything." And try to do everything with great effort and give it your best. Do this with even the smallest of tasks. When you adopt this attitude, excellence will start to become aa habit.
2. **Boosting self-confidence**. Every challenge you have and will go through enhances your personal growth. Lean on past successes in moments of doubt and talk to mentors or coaches when necessary. An outside perspective from the right people can help change your outlook and/or approach to a difficult problem.
3. **Self-talk matters.** Our self-talk shapes our perception of ourselves to the world. It can also change our entire attitude, how we look and feel, and our entire output. By working on positive and empowering internal conversations, we can influence our actions and interactions at the same time of boosting our self-confidence. Try to make it a daily habit to affirm your

# JUST LIVE IT

worth and potential. Look in the mirror and tell yourself how freaking awesome you are!

# Chapter 10

# Be All In

*"Passion is energy. Feel the power that comes from focusing on what excites you."*

**Oprah Winfrey, American host, and television producer**

There is a fine line between casually wandering and trying things out "just to see," and passionately pursuing something you love and are obsessed with. Any person's journey is going to have a lot of twists and turns, many of which are able to deter people from the path, causing them to burn out and give up, in hopes of the next thing working out. When it comes to chasing our dreams, you can't do it half-baked. You're either in it or you're not.

I know, at least in bodybuilding, you're not going to win on stage if you don't give it everything you have. Any person with an enormous amount of success, they didn't get there by not going all in on it. When you give yourself to your goals, the world takes notice, and the universe helps you get there.

## Going the Distance

People have often asked why I go so hard with things I do. When I had my first few businesses, I was going 100 mph, and there was no slowing down. At first, it came from being in survival mode my whole life, so I didn't know any better. Then, after a while, it just became a part of how I operated, because it has helped things work out.

It was interesting to read about P. Diddy during COVID. While people were building new businesses and seeking out opportunities, he said, "If this [COVID] didn't bring the hustle out in you, you ain't got it." I felt that.

If there's a drive in you, and some extreme circumstances, like losing your job, don't bring it out, then it just might not be there. Challenges should amplify your efforts and drive, not extinguish them.

You see, when you're all in on your passions and actually committed to something, it becomes a part of you. This commitment is a two-way street, though. There might be times when it seems you're doing everything you can and pushing as hard as possible, but at a certain point, things have to break. Eventually, the universe will give back and give you certain pushes along the way, helping you get closer and closer to your goals. It might be a little nudge or offering like a new person in your network, a new client, or some other break. But either way, you will get in return what you give to your mission.

What you put out is what you will get back. In fact, when you put all your effort in, you get ten times as much back. Your intentions, the energy you bring, the work you put in, all create ripples that can help shape your reality. If your intention is pure and you put in the effort with all your heart, you will witness returns that exceed your expectations.

I remember once, early in my personal training career, I was behind a lady in the grocery store who didn't have enough money for all of her groceries. The day before, an old client had decided to switch coaches to change things up and see how his progress improved or not. That was totally cool with me—exploring other coaches and seeing what's out there. That client happened to owe me one more payment of a thousand dollars, and I wasn't sure if or when it would show up.

The lady's groceries were about fifty dollars, and I gave her the money to buy all of her groceries and keep what money she had. A couple of days later, an assistant of mine called and told me that the client paid his last installment, but that there was another thousand-dollar payment from him months ago that had never gotten cashed at the bank. So, just like that, I was up two thousand dollars!

I promise you, when you have pure intentions and act on them in ways to help others, you will be blessed in more abundant ways.

## Commitment to Healing

With all this talk about being all in, I think it's only fair to share where my priorities currently lie. Right now, I'm completely immersed in helping people heal from whatever ails them. I decided to quit coaching athletes last year. It was too stressful for me, much more so than when I was competing. As a competitor, I loved it, but it's too hard on my body now to coach other people. One of the last athletes I finished with was Kai Greene to the Olympia on his last 2$^{nd}$ place finish. Of course, there's fulfillment in helping the world I so love and came up in, but I'm called toward a different path now.

I want to help people heal by using my knowledge of nutrition, exercise, lifestyle changes, and mindset shifts. It's been a blessing to see some of the transformations that have happened in front of my very eyes. Few things have filled me with this much joy, and I'm all in on this current mission at hand. When I see someone regain their health, especially after being told they were going to die, it reminds me of why I started all this in the first place. Remember, never forget why you started. It will keep you going at any point along your journey.

To be all in is a lot easier said than done. It will take all of you, but it will reward you more than you think possible. It's the difference between those who dream of it, and those who live out those dreams. There's no halfway. And if you're not ready to give your entire being to your passions, then it might not be the right time, or it might not be the right passion. And those are okay places to be at in life. Very few people ever figure it all out on their first go. But you have to keep trying if you want to chase something bigger than yourself. Try things until you find where your heart truly lies.

Life has a unique way of reflecting back what we put into it. Your efforts, intentions, and integrity matter. Whether you're pursuing a dream, trying to overcome a challenge, or aiming to make a difference, remember to give it everything you have.

In Matthew McConaughey's book, *Green Lights*, he tells the story about the first time he told his dad that he wanted to go to film school. His dad asked him if that's what he really wanted to do, and Matthew told him, "Yes." After a couple seconds of silence, his dad told him, "Don't half-ass it."

JUST LIVE IT

# **Takeaways**

1. **Commitment over casualty.** Success and fulfillment come from an unwavering commitment to your dreams. It doesn't matter if it's a personal project, a job, or a relationship, look at where you stand with any and all of it. If it's important enough to take time out of your day, then give it an honest effort. Give it everything you can.
2. **Reciprocal energy.** The universe has a funny way of reflecting back the energy we put into our endeavors. By giving 100% to what you truly believe in, you'll find that life often rewards you in kind, often in ways you'd never expect.
3. **Passions fuel purpose.** When you're all in on your dreams, they become more than just hobbies or interests. They shape your purpose, guiding you through every up and down with clarity and enthusiasm. Try to pinpoint your passions and let them be the compass guiding your journey.

## Chapter 11

# Money is Important, But It's Not Everything

*"Money is numbers and numbers never end. If it takes money to be happy, your search for happiness will never end."*

**Bob Marley, Jamaican singer, and musician**

Tom Cruise acted in a movie back in the 80s called *The Color of Money.* The premise is that Cruise is a talented protégé in the game of pool, and at a certain point, he has to make a miraculous comeback. There is a scene where he's discussing what he wants from the game with his mentor, and

## JUST LIVE IT

his mentor asks him what he's trying to get out of playing. Cruise responds, "I'm not. I'm gonna win it all." It wasn't just about the money for Cruise's character, but more about the love for the game. He wanted to prove himself in a game that he loved. The money was just a side bonus.

In my particular type of work, as well as many others, people want to talk with the experts. The term "expert" is not one I throw around lightly. It takes years of effort, discipline, trial and error, studying, passion, and a love for the game.

There's a doctor and author whose work I'm a big fan of, Dr. Peter Attia, who's an expert in longevity medicine. He specializes in trying to help people live a longer, healthier, fuller life. He actually just came out with a great book called *Outlive: The Science and Art of Longevity,* outlining some of these longevity principles. He didn't get where he is for the money. He loves this line of work—helping people—and has a passion for the game.

In all my years, the moments that have brought me the most joy and satisfaction weren't necessarily the ones where I earned the most money. It was when I saw genuine growth in those I was helping, when I could make a noticeable difference in the lives of others.

If someone told me I could go back to my health pre-cancer, and all I had to do was give up all the money I have, I'd do it in a heartbeat. Money will come and go, but there are things like your health, memories with loved ones, precious moments that all the money in the world couldn't buy. Let me ask you this: if someone offered you a hundred million dollars today, but you wouldn't wake up the next day, would you take it? Money is only a tool; it's not everything.

## Paying It Forward: Lessons from Battling Cancer

It might seem a bit crazy to read, and every once in a while, it's kind of crazy to think, but if it weren't for my battle with cancer, I'm not sure I would've discovered my newfound love for helping others heal. My love for being the helping hand that pulls people out of the darkness is something that I'm not sure I would've found without my own extreme battles. I learned the proactive and holistic approach to one's health and how to live a more preventative life rather than a reactive one.

Over the years, particularly after my recovery, I've studied and stumbled upon some of the most enlightening and simple-sounding tips for everyday staples. For example, if you're having a migraine or severe headache, it could very well be linked to sodium intake. If you soak your feet in hot water, as hot as you can handle, it could help draw some of that out and relieve your headache.

Muslims seem to have the lowest risk of cancer out of any other culture in the world. There are a handful of theories that might play into this from spices to lack of alcohol and tobacco use, but the one that has some serious weight to it and is the most fascinating to me is fasting. They practice Ramadan, where they go through long periods of time in the day where they fast. Fasting has the potential to starve the potential cancer cells, thus aiding the Muslim community in reducing the risk of cancer.

After my recovery, the demand for my expertise went through the roof. It reached a point where I had to open my own place for a while to keep up with all the demand. I couldn't do it on my own any longer, though. Even then, money wasn't the primary driver. Don't get me wrong; it's nice to have and allows me the freedom to live the life I want, but I did and do these things because I love to do it and purely want to help others. I had athletes who were hungry and dedicated, coming to me who were broke and chasing a dream. A place I knew all too well. They said they couldn't pay my fees for a while. I'd tell them, "Let's get you the win first. We'll talk money later." It was never about the money.

## Investing in Health, Not Just Wealth

I live a blessed life. Even if I could complain, nobody would want to hear it! But seriously, this life has given me more than I could've asked for. And if there's one thing I've learned, it's that your health is your true wealth. If you had all the money in the world and were sick in a hospital bed, then what's the point? The investments you make in your body will never produce returns like you see in the stock market, but it will give you the ability to continue living in a way that doesn't limit you from achieving your dreams, because you'll be able-bodied and healthy to keep chasing. While money can open doors, it's all the intangibles behind your "why" that will make sure you walk through those doors healthy, and with pride.

The next time you're faced with a choice between money and something that genuinely matters to you, truly lights your fire, stop and think about it for a moment. One, do you have to choose one or the other? Yes, money is essential, so cover your bills and make sure you can live. But at the end of the day, you will work harder on your passion than you ever will doing anything else. And with that kind of work ethic, I promise you the money will come. It might be faster, it might be slower, but I promise it will come, and it will be in abundance. At the end of the day, it's not about how much you earn, but how much you give, love, and live.

## **Takeaways**

1. **Value beyond wealth.** While money plays a crucial role in today's society, remember its limitations. It will always come and go. It can buy things and temporary comfort, but it cannot buy love, happiness, or precious

# JUST LIVE IT

time spent with those you love. Always weigh the monetary gain against the intangibles that make the world go round.

2. **Proactive health is the game.** Investing in your health, both mental and physical, is the best interment you can make in yourself. Money becomes insignificant if you're too sick to do anything with it. Make sure you take proactive measures in your health to ensure you live a long, healthy life where you're able to do all the things you want to in this lifetime.

3. **Pay it forward.** Giving, whether in terms of knowledge, time, or resources, often brings more fulfillment than accumulating wealth. But if you do pay it forward and give those things to others, the wealth will show up on your doorstep. The act of helping someone with zero expectation in return generates a feeling that no dollar amount ever can. It also emphasizes the type of integrity and character you have.

# Chapter 12

# Prioritizing Health and Body Care

*"How we care for our body is the most important piece of knowledge we can learn. Because without health, what do we really have?"*

**Leonardo da Vinci, Italian polymath**

    With my love for health and helping others, I wanted to include some daily practices and rituals that I subscribe to. I think it's also fair to illuminate on some things I see wrong within the healthcare and drug system and provide some simple things that most people could do without much concern. And they are things that might start to have a pretty quick impact on your health and how you feel.

Take things as you will, do your own research, and consult with any physician of yours if necessary. Again, these are just some things I'm a big proponent of and that have worked for me as well as others.

## Nature's Pharmacy

We have some of the most natural healing components at our disposal, and they're completely free—sunlight, fresh air, and the ground under your feet. Dr. Andrew Huberman is very bullish about getting morning sunlight in your eyes. Now, you don't need to stare directly into the sun, but getting some morning sun exposure can help set your circadian rhythm and prime your body for the day.

While you're outside, go out there barefoot and practice some grounding. I did this every day during my battle with cancer. Doing so can help reduce stress, shift the nervous system from sympathetic to parasympathetic (helps drop cortisol), speed wound healing, and also normalize our circadian rhythm. The earth can give us a lot, so why not take advantage and do some good for your body and overall health?

# Fasting and the Alkaline Diet

We touched on the power of fasting earlier, but it has a lot of benefits: regulate blood sugar, improve hormone balances, starve diseases, such as cancer, improve sleep, and cognitive abilities. I typically try to do a sixteen-hour fast, with an eight-hour window to eat. I'd recommend doing your best to still get your required number of calories in that eight-hour window, but don't force-feed yourself.

The alkaline diet is also a useful tool that I'm still doing every day and have done with lots of clients to help heal their ailments. I mentioned before that during my battle with cancer, the alkaline diet helped me heal faster than anyone else getting similar treatments. Had I been able to do this diet before going into my first couple surgeries where they removed my prostate and bladder, I don't think they would've needed to do that.

The alkaline diet is basically a raw vegan diet, consisting of fruits and vegetables, reducing meat intake, no processed foods, no alcohol, and keeping things as natural as possible. The idea is to maintain the body's ideal pH levels and help reduce inflammation and disease.

## Cannabis: Plant Medicine, to My Surprise

As mentioned before, when I was going through all the surgeries, the doctors put me in a bunch of opioids. After a short while, those drugs started giving me more grief than relief. I had the wildest suicidal thoughts, which I never had before taking those pills. And since getting off of them, I haven't had them since.

I started eating gummies that had both THC and CBD in them, both cannabinoids found to show a lot of promise within various health benefits. Those are only two out of a hundred cannabinoids within the cannabis plants. There are plenty of non-psychoactive cannabinoids that are being reported and shown to offer a lot of aid to a handful of ailments and conditions.

Federally, a lot of cannabis products are legal, mainly the non-psychoactive ones. So, states are starting to come around and be more open to plant alternatives. I still take them and haven't touched an opioid since.

## Big Pharma

I'll never say that we don't need Western medicine or traditional doctors, procedures, and certain prescription drugs. There are a lot of good things that come with Western medicine, and a lot of people who get help from such.

However, it is hard to imagine that the big pharmaceutical companies are not in this just for the money. With what some of these drugs do to people, how addictive they can be, and with the working alternatives to them, it seems there is another agenda. It pains me that many giants in the pharmaceutical industry seem more inclined to profit than to heal. Their skepticism about alternative medicine, particularly cannabis, is laughable.

Just in 2021, Pfizer bought a CBG company. CBG is a cannabinoid called cannabigerol, which has been known for its anti-inflammatory properties, but especially its ability to help improve gut health. They bought a whole company dedicated to one cannabinoid, and hardly anyone knows about it. My fear is that the pharma companies will speak out against cannabis products enough to halt their momentum, buy up what they can, be all for them, and monopolize (and ruin) that industry. If CBG stops benefiting folks the way it does now, we'll know why, along with the true intentions.

## Water: Life's Elixir

We all know it's important to stay hydrated, but just how hydrated should we be? A simple formula that I like to give to people is to take your body weight and multiply it by .6, and that is the number of ounces of water you should drink each day. However, if you drink coffee, you must replace each cup of coffee with a cup of water. Coffee is a diuretic, so you need to replace it with water.

I also like to start my day by squeezing a whole lemon into eight ounces of water in the morning, on an empty stomach. It can help flush toxins, balance your body's pH level, and can even give you an energy boost. Medical Medium is another trusted source of information who advises on about half a lemon worth of lemon juice, but I would like to add a bit more. It can also be a good friend to your liver.

## Move Often – We're Supposed To

Regular movement and exercise have been proven time and time again to greatly improve overall health and biomarkers. We're not meant to be sedentary creatures, yet that's how most of our society lives their lives and has done so for years. Our ancestors were always on the move, hunting, gathering, building, and always having something to do and somewhere to go. Even simple walks and stretching sessions can do the body wonders.

There's so much around us that we can use at our disposal to improve our lives. However, there's no one-size-fits-all to one's health and wellness. It takes plenty of research, trial and error, and finding what resonates with your mind, body, and spirit. Whether it's the food you eat, the medicines you take, or grounding and exercising, make choices that are preventative and that honor your body.

# Takeaways

1. **Power of proactive health.** Your body is the most intricate and valuable machine you own. It's rented. Take proactive health measures, like starting your day with lemon water, eating a natural diet, and getting proper sleep and regular exercise. These practices can help build a foundation that can set you up for a lifelong time of health and happiness.
2. **Question everything.** The pharmaceutical industry, like any other business, aims to profit. But their aim to profit is above their aim to heal. Always do your research, ask questions, and be open to alternative therapies and treatments. My positive experience with cannabis products underscores the importance of keeping an open mind and staying informed.
3. **Nature's healing touch.** From grounding to getting morning sun in your eyes, nature can offer a wealth of therapeutic practices. It's crucial to incorporate daily habits, like grounding and sun gazing, as they benefit the body, mind, and soul.

# Chapter 13

# Guru

**(A Deeper Dive into My Legacy)**

---

*"The two most important days in your life are the day you are born and the day you find out why."*

**Mark Twain, American writer, and humorist**

Lately, I've found myself reflecting on my life quite a bit. The ups, the downs, lessons learned, and all my blessings. It's an overwhelming yet deeply humbling experience to look back on everything and see how far I've come, the people I've helped, and those who have helped me. As I type this last chapter, preparing to close out my journey to you in its most vivid and rawest form to date, I can't help but feel a rush of nostalgia, pride, humility, and immense gratitude.

# Guru

*The Guru Farrah* is an upcoming documentary that I've been working on. It's an account of my entire life, journey, and legacy. It will have stories and testimonies from champions who I have trained, the health battles I've faced and, most importantly, the lessons I want to leave behind for others. And while this book has been my heart poured out on paper, this documentary will be my soul in motion.

The camera can capture a different experience to my story that words can't always convey. It'll show the blood, sweat, and tears from those I've trained, myself, the people with terminal diseases who finally let go of them, and the discipline and determination in all the people whom I've been fortunate enough to come across in my life. All of these warriors became more than just my friends; they became my family.

Within these testimonies, you'll hear stories of resilience, and stories that will hopefully inspire you to face your challenges with courage and determination. I hope they push you to move past your fears and any bumps in the road, and face everything head-on. My health battles, particularly the fight against cancer, have been a core moment within my story. In the documentary, you'll witness the depth of these battles. You'll see that every day was a lesson, even the hard ones, and ones that I had to learn to get to where I am today.

# JUST LIVE IT

I've clearly been pretty vocal about my discoveries in alternative medicine, the pharmaceutical industry's games, and the wonders of simple, holistic health practices. The film will continue highlighting all these aspects of my approach to health and wellness in an effort to broaden the horizons for many who might be seeking answers just like I was.

This book, the documentary, and every moment I've lived are dedicated to those who believe, fight, and love unconditionally. In this world, where the horizon is vast and the paths are many, it's essential to know that every moment counts. I hope my story, in its entirety, reminds you to live with purpose, cherish simple joys and, above all, to never stop learning and growing. Remember, every champion, every guru, starts with a single step, a single punch, a single dream. Keep dreaming, keep fighting, and keep believing.

## **<u>Takeaways</u>**

1. **Leaving a legacy.** It's not just about being remembered but the meaningful impact and inspiration you leave behind. I encourage you to start thinking of what you can leave behind for loved ones to help inspire them to continue doing good work of their own for others.
2. **Everyone has a story.** Deep dive into your own personal journey and find the lessons and growth

within your experiences. Even in the struggles, there are blessings in disguise. Although they might not reveal themselves to you as quickly as others, never neglect that they're there.

3. **Stay authentic.** Never change who you are deep down. Sharing genuine testimonies and stories can help inspire others, serving as powerful reminders to embrace vulnerability and authenticity in life.

JUST LIVE IT

# Join Our Community

---

In the heart of every individual lies the potential for greatness.

If you're reading this and thinking that you have another version of yourself still undiscovered and the time is now to get started on this journey, we have a gift for you.

In this book we are revealing a special opportunity to follow my workouts, meal plans and mindset recordings as if I was traveling with you inside your phone.

My workouts are not a simple PDF but a customized program based on my dumbbell approach to training. My plans evolve with you, pushing your boundaries and fostering growth to prevent stagnation. If you have any injuries, let me know when you sign up and I'll remind you to go easy on exercises that affect the affected muscle group.

This program is delivered inside my own convenient mobile app for Apple and Android so you can access it any time. Having said that, it isn't just a tool; it's really a gateway to transformation, designed with the precision of a champion's regimen and the care of a personalized mentorship.

## GEORGE FARAH, PHD

As you know I am known for my unique approach to nutrition. No garbage food. Clean, real food. As part of my nutrition program I customize meal plans and tailor them to your unique nutritional needs and preferences, whether you're exploring veganism, keto, or any dietary style. Sticking to the plan is the most important thing. I will create a plan for you and update it monthly, but I don't want to update it if you're not using it.

Beyond physical transformation, this program offers an immersive journey into mental, emotional, and spiritual well-being, featuring exclusive content to inspire and guide. With my guidance, you're not just training; you're embarking on a journey of self-discovery and empowerment. Mindset is the foundation, with programs designed to reshape your perspective on discipline and motivation, pivotal for lasting change.

## JUST LIVE IT

    This is more than an app; it's a community, a philosophy, and a new beginning. Welcome to a new era of training, where champions are made, one day, one meal, one mindset shift at a time. Welcome to George Farah's world, where your potential is limitless, and every day is an opportunity to surpass the ordinary.

To join our community and begin your transformation, scan this QR code and get started!

Made in United States
North Haven, CT
19 April 2024

51542652R00075